INFECTED

SECRETS FROM THE MEDICAL UNDERGROUND
How You Can Prevent and Treat Any Infection

RALPH LA GUARDIA M.D.

WRITERS REPUBLIC L.L.C.
515 Summit Ave. Unit R1
Union City, NJ 07087, USA

Website: *www.writersrepublic.com*
Hotline: *1-877-656-6838*
Email: *info@writersrepublic.com*

Ordering Information:
Quantity sales. Special discounts are available on quantity purchases by corporations, associations, and others. For details, contact the publisher at the address above.

Library of Congress Control Number: 2021922758
ISBN-13:   978-1-64620-946-0   [Paperback Edition]
                    978-1-63728-693-7   [Digital Edition]

Rev. date: 11/19/2021

A Word of Caution to the Reader

TABLE OF CONTENTS

Chapter Five

Chapter Eight

Chapter Nine

DEDICATION

First and foremost, I dedicate this book to my Lord and Savior Jesus Christ. Only through your grace and blessings can our bodies and mind ever be truly healed. You have blessed my life over and over again, and continue to do so in countless ways. I am truly grateful knowing that I am not worthy of your continual love and grace, yet you still continue to bestow it upon me. For that and so many other reasons, I will forever be eternally grateful and will always love and adore you. You have proven over and over again that miracle shall follow miracle and wonders shall never cease.

To my amazing wife, Lynne, you have enriched and blessed my life in so many ways since the day I met you. You are my soul mate, the love of my life, and my best friend. You seem to have an inexhaustible stream of skills and previously hidden talents that never cease to amaze me. You are an endless fountain of love and support, and you give 110 percent every day to everything you do and to everyone who has contact with you. You are truly the sunshine of my life, and I am blessed by God to have you as my wife. That being said, I am not buying you any more horses. I liked it better when you played tennis.

To my deceased son, Marcus. I will never ever get over your death. Part of my heart light was extinguished that day, never to be relit. My only consolation is that we will be reunited again someday in heaven, and every day will be like our annual father-son days we both loved so much.

To my rescue dog, Bear, you are the best doggie ever. You weaseled your way into everyone's heart, including the heart of my ninety-one-year-old mother, Mary, who for the first time learned how truly special dogs are and has fallen head over heels for "her baby." For that and countless other reasons, you will always have a special place in my heart.

To my office manager, Jennifer Sonstrom, thank you for printing the endless stream of articles I forward to you daily. It was an immense help to me. That does not mean I am giving you a raise!

And a special thanks to Gary Gile. You are a great friend, an outstanding handyman, a patriot, and an outstanding IT guy. Thank God for your patience, endless prodding, or I would still be on chapter 5. And with your help, I know I will finish my fourth book, "*The Collagen Cure*", this winter. I truly appreciate all the help you provided that made this book possible, and I will be forever grateful.

INTRODUCTION

You have in your hands the most comprehensive, up-to-date book on mostly unknown, hence the designation: "secret" ways to prevent and treat any infection. These methods have arisen from what I like to call *the Medical Underground* .

What I mean by that is the informal worldwide group of physicians and medical researchers who are pioneering, innovative, very effective methods to both prevent and treat all kinds of infections that are not currently recognized or approved by mainstream medicine. These are doctors who have not accepted medical dogma and are thinking outside of the box, finding new, exciting, and oftentimes very effective methods of treating their patients.

Many of these treatments are old remedies that have been repurposed for treating current diseases. They have been around for decades, and many are designated GRAS (generally recognized as safe) by the FDA. Others are innovative combinations of plant-based medicines, minerals, trace elements, and vitamins. Others are over-the-counter medications used in new and exciting ways, such as baking soda and hydrogen peroxide to name a few. Sometimes, old drugs are effectively repurposed for new diseases.

Most of these treatments are not patentable by pharmaceutical companies, and thus they have not invested in expensive clinical trials that would prove their usefulness. Despite this, the medical underground trudges on, oftentimes doing their own clinical studies from their private practices.

Being outside of the medical mainstream is oftentimes punished by the powers that be, but these brave physicians continue their work despite ridicule and condemnation by colleagues who will not accept any treatment that is outside of the current dogma and not accompanied by volumes of clinical studies on thousands of patients. That will never happen with the vast majority of these treatments since without the ability to patent them, they cannot be sold for a profit from pharmaceutical companies.

I and many other medical underground physicians take our Hippocratic Oath very seriously. For us, there are no lengths that we will not go to in search of cures for our sick patients. In my own case, I have spent my entire career searching for these obscure, unknown cures for my patients. I have spent most of my life reading countless books and thousands of articles in medical journals from all over the world.

I have written two earlier books that have been widely acclaimed in the circles of the medical underground, *The Doomsday Book of Medicine* and *The Bible of Alternative Medicine*. *The Doomsday Book of Medicine* has become a cult classic among preppers, filling a serious gap in the literature on medical preparedness.

In this age of COVID-19 and other serious infections, I have turned my attention to their prevention and treatment. I find it incredibly fulfilling to empower my readers with methods they can employ to improve their health.

The public is hankering for ways they can prevent infections and maintain their health. This book will provide them with all the tools they need to both prevent and treat any infection they may encounter, all without prescription medications. My hope is that you will enjoy reading this book as much as I enjoyed writing it and that it will provide you with all the tools you need to both prevent and treat any infection.

Best regards,
Dr. Ralph La Guardia

CHAPTER ONE

WHERE DO COLDS, FLU, AND CORONAVIRUSES ORIGINATE?

The coronavirus is not new as a pathogen or disease-causing virus. In a typical cold and flu season, there are about two hundred different viruses that infect humans. Of this two hundred, approximately 15 percent, or thirty, are coronaviruses.

The vast majority of the viruses that cause our colds and flu are rhinoviruses. There are also influenza viruses and adenoviruses, followed by a smattering of lesser-known viruses.

The problem with these viruses, especially the flu virus, is that they constantly mutate. This constant mutation leads to changes in the protein antigens found on the surface of these viruses. This is known as antigenic drift.

When you are infected with a virus of any type, you develop antibodies that protect you from subsequent infections with the same virus. Once antigenic drift occurs and the surface proteins change, then the antibodies no longer recognize it; and hence, we have no immunity to the new virus.

That is the reason you never develop immunity to the flu and need a different vaccine every year.

Why does the flu and other viruses like coronavirus always seem to come out of China and other places in Asia?

The world reservoir for flu virus is in the wild bird population. For the coronavirus it is found in bats. People underestimate the number of bats of different species there are worldwide. Bats comprise 25 percent of all mammals!

In Asia, farmers raise both ducks and pigs together. That is not the practice in other parts of the world. This is the reason that the flu always originates from Asia.

Humans usually cannot catch the flu from a bird, but a pig can. And you guessed it—the virus can be transmitted from a pig to a human. Thus the wild birds interact with the domestic ducks, infecting them, and they in turn pass it on to the pigs and from them to us.

Since these viruses, especially the flu, arise in Asia, the CDC sends teams to Asia months before our flu season begins and finds the three most common types and produces the annual flu vaccine.

By the way, it is insanity to think that calling a virus that originates in China Chinese is racist. That is typical political correctness gone wild. Viruses are frequently named for their geographic origins. For example: West Nile Virus, Zika virus (the Zika forest of Uganda), Middle East Respiratory Syndrome (MERS), etc.

The coronavirus that is presently causing unprecedented damage to the world economy originated in Wuhan, China. The party line that mainstream media is spewing so obediently is that its origin is currently thought to have been from a wild animal market.

These markets are common all over China, where they sell snakes, rodents, pandas, and many types of bats. Apparently, the Chinese like eating bats. They also have a festival celebrating the summer solstice in Yulin, Guangxi, China, where dogs are eaten! Personally, I think that dogs are the greatest animals on the planet, and I have three that I adore; so for me seeing Labradors, hounds, and boxers on meat hooks is absolutely disgusting. However, I digress.

It appears that someone got infected from these wild bats, which harbor coronaviruses of many types. That leap to human infection was the result of either a mutation of a known coronavirus or from a new or novel coronavirus, perhaps one man-made in a lab, which seems the most likely scenario.

There is also mounting evidence that this was a virus that was man-made in that lab and either escaped accidentally or intentionally. The jury is still out on which one. The actual lab in Wuhan was doing "gain of function" research on coronaviruses.

What *gain of function* means is that scientists manipulate the virus to make it more infectious to humans. For example, they make it easier to attach to our lungs' cells after we inhale it. This newfound affinity for lung cells will weaponize a respiratory virus, making it much more contagious to humans.

The theory is that the scientists can then learn ways to block these novel viruses with vaccines to protect us in the future. Weak theory at best, with the potential for absolute disaster if something goes wrong, like you might cause a pandemic that cripples the entire world! That is why this type of research was outlawed in the United States.

Apparently, recently released e-mails of Dr. Anthony Fauci showed that, incredibly, he was instrumental in continuing this research in China of, all places; and China is a country absolutely obsessed with our destruction. Hmmm, what genius thought that was a good idea?

From the beginning, one had to be willing to ignore the obvious mountain of evidence pointing to a lab origin—the evidence actually includes Chinese virologist defectors who told of it originating there—and accept the ridiculous theory that this came from a wet market across town.

Once President Trump correctly opined that he thought it was from the coronavirus virology lab in Wuhan, the mainstream media, in their anti-all-things-Trump hysteria went ballistic, mocking him as a "conspiracy theorist" and went all in on the wet-market-infected-bat nonsense. Anyone who dared think otherwise was openly ridiculed as antiscience as well as being racist against the Chinese.

Currently, there are three companies manufacturing COVID-19 vaccines, Moderna and Pfizer, both of which make an mRNA vaccine, and Johnson and Johnson, which makes a DNA vaccine. The mRNA vaccines require two injections approximately three weeks apart. The DNA vaccine is one injection and done. As of the time of this book's writing, approximately 180 million Americans have been vaccinated at least once. There is a "delta variant" spreading throughout the world, after originating in India, there is an alpha variant from England, and the beta variant from South Africa. The most recent count on the number of variants of COVID-19 currently stands around four thousand

and is naturally on the rise. Despite what the Biden administration bloviates about, this is not a pandemic fueled by variants arising in the unvaccinated. On the contrary, the variants arise in the vaccinated. The reason is that in the unvaccinated, there is little to no selective pressure on the virus. In the vaccinated, the virus has to evade their immune system, which already has been primed by the vaccine. This creates great selective pressure on the virus and hence the profusion of variants.

Many of the patients getting infected with the delta variant have already been fully vaccinated. The actual percentages vary from country to country, but in some places, they are the majority of the new COVID-19 cases. It appears that this vaccine fails the two criteria of a vaccine: to prevent you from contracting the virus and to prevent its transmission. It does appear to decrease the severity of the disease and thus its mortality, but at what price? This naturally begs the question: if by definition this is not a vaccine, then what is it? It is gene therapy, where the vaccine permanently alters our DNA, and you are still transmitting the virus as well.

The United States government has a system for reporting adverse events from vaccines. It is known as VAERS: Vaccine Adverse Events Reporting System. Doctors report adverse events to VAERS, and it is compiled there. So far, the numbers are very disturbing, to say the least.

Number of adverse events reported: 675,591

Deaths: 14,506

Hospitalizations: 58,440

Urgent care visits: 77,519

Doctor's office visits: 106,184

Anaphylaxis: 5,783

Bell's palsy: 7,911

Miscarriages: 1,757

Heart attacks: 6,422

Myocarditis: 5,371

Permanently disabled: 18,439

Thrombocytopenia or low platelets: 2,910

Life-threatening reaction: 14,594

Severe allergic reaction: 27,336

Shingles: 7,810

Call me crazy, but this is one scary list of adverse reactions to the COVID-19 vaccines. Yes, you can make the argument that it is due to the massive numbers of vaccinated Americans. However, in 1976, when the swine flu broke out at Fort Dix, New Jersey, we began mass vaccinations, and over fifty patients developed Guillain-Barré syndrome and thirty or so died, and the vaccination program was deemed too dangerous and was halted. "Hmmm," you say, scratching your chin, "why is it so different now?" Good question, grasshopper. I don't know the answer. I do know that it should give any rational person pause.

The vaccine also does not prevent you from transmitting the virus. Those two reasons alone make me wonder about the usefulness of such a vaccine. That coupled with the novel mechanism of action, with its unknown long-term side effects, really should give one pause.

Now if you are in your eighties, the benefits probably outweigh the potential negatives, but that is a discussion that a doctor and a patient should have, without the intrusion of state or federal laws, in my humble opinion.

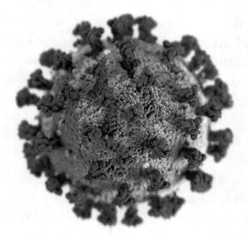

The coronavirus family is so named for its appearance under an electron microscope, where it has many surface proteins protruding out on spikes, giving it the appearance of a crown, which in Latin is called *corona*.

COVID-19 means coronavirus disease of 2019. Ironically, it was named on the very last day of 2019. Otherwise, it would have added to the infamy of 2020, which for many was the absolute worst year of their lives, including myself with the death of my beloved son, Marcus.

To further complicate matters, COVID-19 is caused by a specific type of coronavirus called SARS-CoV-2 or severe acute respiratory syndrome coronavirus 2.

SARS-1, as you might recall, was a very dangerous outbreak during the 2002–2003 flu season. It had a fatality rate of 9.6 percent, much higher than the current death rate for COVID-19, which hovers around 0.028 percent. In actuality, it is probably even lower than that, since the thirty-eight million flu cases in 2019 essentially disappeared once COVID-19 reared its ugly head, in addition to which it is believed that a large number of people get sick with COVID-19 and are not seen by a health-care provider due to a paucity of symptoms. Both of those factors would drive down the current COVID-19 death rate.

As of the writing of this book, it was similar to the seasonal flu, and is very likely to drop even lower due to the massive number of undiagnosed people.

I have a large primary care practice here in the country in Connecticut. I see countless patients who have cold, flu, bronchitis, and pneumonia. I have no way currently to distinguish COVID-19 from the others, hence these patients are going undiagnosed. Only the most severe patients with fevers and respiratory failure are presenting to local hospitals all over the country and getting diagnosed.

This falsely skewers the numbers in favor of a higher death rate. I do have testing available to me, and it is becoming increasingly easier to test patients.

Outbreaks of deadly epidemics of corona and flu viruses occur like clockwork every few years. We occasionally dodge the bullet of a very deadly outbreak as we did in 2012 with the MERS (Middle East Respiratory Syndrome).

MERS is a coronavirus that apparently had its reservoir in camels. Since camels come in close contact with humans in the Middle East (no snide comments), that was a natural place from which to jump to humans, as it did in 2012. MERS has an amazingly high fatality rate of 34.4 percent! That is incredibly fatal.

To keep that in perspective, the Spanish flu of 1918 had a fatality rate of 2.5 percent and was estimated to kill over fifty million people worldwide. It was severe enough that it ended World War I. The reason was that unlike most influenza or flu outbreaks, this targeted young people in the prime of their lives, in their twenties and thirties.

The old and the young were spared. The presumption is that the old had to have been infected years before with a flu virus strain that was close enough to the Spanish flu that their immune system was still effective in protecting them. It had to be at least thirty-plus years ago since the majority of the victims of the Spanish flu were under thirty.

It is not clear why the very young were spared. One theory says the immune systems of both the young and the old were not as robust as adults between twenty and forty. Ironically, a robust immune system caused the release of large amounts of inflammatory cytokines, called a cytokine storm, which kills its victims.

There is also a theory that huge doses of aspirin were used, which led to hemorrhaging and pulmonary edema (fluid in the lungs), thus spiking the mortality rates of the Spanish flu. In other words, the cure in this case was worse than the disease!

Thus at the height of World War I, when millions of young men were being hoarded together in training camps and on crowded troop ships, it became the perfect environment for the spread of infection. It was so deadly that sometimes, nurses or doctors treating patients would start their shifts without symptoms and become ill and die within twelve hours!

It was the worst epidemic since the bubonic plague, or the Black Death, of the Middle Ages, which purportedly killed a third of Europe. The plague came in waves about a century apart. Consequently, no one had any immunity, and it repeatedly ripped thru these virgin populations.

The plague typically killed between 30 and 90 percent of those infected within about ten days. Unlike the flu and coronavirus, the plague was caused by a bacterium, *Yersinia pestis*. As you can see, it was much deadlier than any of the worst viruses we historically have experienced.

The Spanish flu did the same thing, coming in three successive waves. However, these were annual waves. Eventually, almost everyone alive had developed protective antibodies and thus were immune to a repeat infection, and hence the virus ran out of hosts and petered out.

As with other infections we have studied, the Spanish flu most likely came from an area in France, where large supplies of pigs and poultry were kept near each other to feed the millions of troops fighting World War I. The theory is that wild birds infected the poultry, they infected the pigs; and from the pigs, it crossed over to infect the human population.

Wartime conditions and poverty, with its malnutrition and overcrowded, unhygienic living conditions all contributed to both the rapid spread and the lethality of this flu.

Looking at the photo below, you will immediately notice that half of the soldiers are not wearing their cloth masks, and they are massed together in large, overcrowded wards. There is no social distancing, and primitive hygiene is being practiced. All these factors facilitated the rapid spread of the virus.

That being said, there is no credible scientific studies showing that social distancing does anything at all. The six-foot rule is absolutely arbitrary, but everyone ran with it. Without a doubt, people huddled together in very close proximity will facilitate viral transmission. I am simply disputing the six-foot nonsense that people freak about, thinking somehow that they are screwed if you are within five feet of them!

Masks are also almost completely ineffective at stopping viral transmission. Incredibly, nobody has asked Dr. Fauci the obvious question: if surgical masks and cloth masks work so well to prevent viral transmission, why are they wearing space suits with fully enclosed pressurized helmets, etc., instead of the face masks?

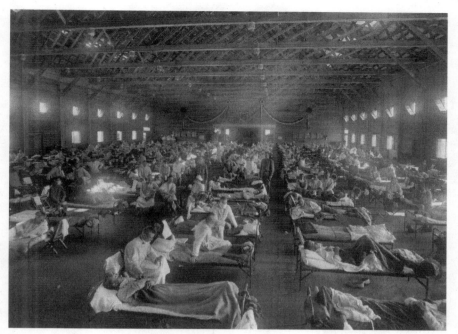

American soldiers infected with the Spanish flu from Fort Riley, Kansas, at a hospital ward at Camp Funston during WWI.

Viruses are not very well understood by the general public. They are fascinating in their behavior. A virus that is extremely lethal like MERS has a difficult time becoming a pandemic. The reason is that the patient gets so sick that they are immediately bedridden and die shortly thereafter.

From the virus's viewpoint, this is an evolutionary dead end since the virus dies with the host. An ideal situation for the virus is to have a long incubation period, during which time the host (patient) is spewing millions of viral particles that are able to infect many other patients.

In short, the virus wants to acquire as much "market share" among the general population as possible, thus guaranteeing its survival. For that reason, it is very much in the virus's self-interest to evolve into a more contagious but less lethal variant of itself. And that is exactly what happens.

They are touting it as being more lethal and even spreads among children, which the current COVID-19 does not do (unlike the flu).

In 2020, nineteen19 children died of COVID-19 in the entire United States, none of whom were in good health.

Compare this to 2019, during which 180 children died of the flu, almost ten times the number of COVID-19. Why on earth are we closing the schools for COVID-19 when we didn't for the flu and nothing happened?

The current hysteria over COVID-19, in my opinion, is totally unwarranted. I believe there will be a serious pandemic that is real and very lethal, but it is not COVID-19.

I cannot imagine that the economic and political devastation unleashed by this relatively benign virus has not been lost on the leaders in China, Russia, Iran, and North Korea to name a few of the bad actors who would love to take down the United States and other Western democracies.

I believe that they will unleash a more serious biological warfare agent on us at some time in the near future. It costs next to nothing to produce and has so much potential for incredible harm, thus making it too irresistible for them. Do you think they are doing all this gain of function weaponization of viruses to develop vaccines for mankind?

You need to wake up and get your act together. This was not a onetime freak event. It was very likely planned, that is why I wrote this book. Pandemic 2.0 is just around the corner, and I want to help as many people as I can prepare themselves for the inevitable.

Hence the importance of a book like this for your very survival and the survival of your family and your community. No other book on the market will teach you how to not only boost your immune system to shield yourself from all types of diseases but also in the unlikely event that you contract an infection. This book will be your personal guide on how to annihilate it quickly and effectively.

Many of the therapies you will learn to utilize in this book are not known by the vast majority of physicians. Doctors like myself, who practice integrative medicine—that is combining the best of traditional medicine along with alternative and complementary medical treatments—have been on the front lines of the medical underground developing novel ways of treating viral and bacterial infections of all kinds.

This can all be accomplished without the use of prescription pharmaceuticals, which in the event of a new pandemic will likely either be unavailable or ineffective. Pandemic 2.0 will make this book worth its weight in gold.

CHAPTER TWO

BUILD THE WALL

Why doesn't everyone get the flu or coronavirus when it is "passing through" the population?

The answer to that question is, it totally depends on your immune system. The stronger your immunity, the more readily it fights off infections.

Think of your immune system as a wall. The stronger your immunity, the higher the wall; and conversely, the weaker your immunity, the lower the wall. Any invading microorganism such as bacteria and viruses need to be strong enough to climb right up that wall to the top and over into our bodies.

Conventional medicine relies almost exclusively on offense. They rarely consider the height of the wall. They would rather have kick-ass troops on the inside of the wall that hopefully will live up to their name and wipe out any invading bacteria or virus. They are essentially fighting a war against invading microorganisms that is all offense, with no defense at all.

From thirty-seven years in practice, I know that patients do infinitely better with disease prevention rather than even the best treatments. But that is rarely the way medicine is practiced. Doctors are well trained and well-intentioned but are generally very overworked especially in the trenches of primary care.

In my country office, for example, I see everything from a stroke, accidental gunshot, heart attack, or chainsaw injury to rashes, sore throats, blocked ears, and psychological problems that run the entire gamut. Consequently, most primary care docs wind up spending the vast majority of their time "putting out fires" and addressing the endless barrage of problems that flow into their offices. Prevention becomes the loser, hence most patients have no defensive game.

I, on the other hand, think that building a strong immunity or higher wall is a better strategy. Not only that but the treatments I utilize are full of beneficial side effects, unlike most current pharmaceuticals.

I am, however, originally from New Jersey; thus I grew up having to be practical. So I am not averse to using traditional pharmaceuticals as a "backup army" to stop any microbial invaders who might make it over the wall.

But that is not the point of this book, which is to teach you what you need to build your own immune wall, shielding your body from infection. You must look at this as a war and you need to fight it to win. Build that wall, your body will thank you and reward you with good health, making you impervious to most infections.

Let this one fact sink into your soul: the only time you get any illness, including COVID-19, is when it overcomes your immune system! That is the only way you get it. We will revisit that concept later in this chapter.

Young adults have the strongest immune systems, and women are stronger than men. Yes, my little snowflakes, the horror! I did say there were only two sexes. Get over it! There are only two, and only you "woke" fools think otherwise. However, I digress.

The presumptive reason for the difference between the sexes is that women carry fetuses, and thus natural selection favors women with more robust immunity. Those women would give birth to more children that survive pregnancy, thus passing on those genes.

Young children have immature immune systems that are not totally developed. As they grow, so does the vigor of their immunity. Immune strength is the reason why the annual flu kills primarily the very young and the very old.

The only other people it kills are those with compromised immune systems, such as AIDS or cancer patients as well as those with multiple illnesses that combine to diminish their immune vigor.

The body's immune system is aided by other barriers to infection that act to reduce the load of any pathogen reaching it. Each of these barriers contribute to the ultimate height of your immunity. The more robust these other barriers to infection are, the greater your "resistance."

Here are some of the building blocks your body uses to build up its wall of immunity.

SKIN

Your skin acts as a physical barrier that germs must cross to infect us. It covers your entire body surface and is our largest organ. The skin weighs in at eight pounds and measures twenty-two square feet in area! It works wonderfully until it is cut or burnt, which creates openings in the skin wall. That is why burns and wounds become infected; the germs entering can evade the first line of defense—the skin's continuous barrier or wall.

Once past the skin, the body's immune system is the last line of defense. Once the immune system is overwhelmed you get a local infection where the skin was broken. If the infection is bad enough, it will spread at first into the adjacent tissues.

Eventually, if unimpeded, it will invade into your blood, spreading to other areas. This is known as sepsis or blood poisoning. If your body is unable to mount an effective counterattack to defeat these invaders, it will disseminate all through your body and eventually kill you.

Your skin has a method to "do its thing," such as sweat. Sweat serves to enhance your immunity. Sweat is remarkably similar in composition to human blood plasma, but with certain components retained by the body and not excreted.

Sweating is another interesting mechanism our bodies have for maintaining their internal body temperature. Only humans, other primates, horses, and some breeds of cattle use this mechanism. The body produces sweat that evaporates on our skin and thus helps rid it of excessive heat and at the same time moisturizing it.

Sweat glands cover your entire body surface, except for your nipples, lips, and areas of your groin. They are also concentrated in certain areas such as your axillae (armpits), soles, palms, and your face. They are controlled by your nervous system.

Remember the last time you were questioned by someone in authority and you began to have sweaty palms? Or when you were supposedly out with the girls and you came home really late and your husband asked you where you were all night? You little hussy...however, I digress.

Once again, the human body often gets multiple benefits from any action it does, including sweating. Besides cooling your body by evaporation, sweat also contains other components such as salts, many minerals, lactate, and urea. The primary minerals are sodium, potassium, calcium, and magnesium as well as a bunch of trace elements. Thus through its chemical composition, sweat has both antibacterial and antifungal properties, further enhancing our skin immunity.

One of the earliest mentioning of sweating by physicians was among the Greeks over two thousand years ago. They used to lick an infant's skin to test if it tasted salty. If so, they would immediately know that this infant would not live long due to cystic fibrosis. Who needs Quest?

Sweating also helps our bodies eliminate harmful toxins such as arsenic, cadmium, lead, mercury, BPA (bisphenol A, which is a by-product of the production of plastics and resins, phthalates, which are used in the production of many PVC plastic products as well as many personal-care items).

Saunas have been utilized for centuries to induce sweating to help rid our bodies of these and many other toxins. Currently, there are both traditional saunas and near-infrared saunas, which are both very good at detoxification.

The skin also releases oils that have dual functions. They act to lubricate the skin, but they also are both antibacterial and antifungal. As if that wasn't enough, the skin also has specialized cells called Langerhans cells, which are macrophages ("big eaters" in Greek). Macrophages get their name from the fact that once they identify a target, they engulf it completely and ingest it. Macrophages are found throughout the skin and in the lining of the respiratory and urogenital tracts.

How cool is that. The skin is ready for fungi, bacteria, and anything else that might try to invade, besides being a huge mechanical barrier. You've got to love the unbelievable design of our bodies; I have been studying it my entire adult life, and I am still in awe. The skin is also aided by an army of microorganisms that coat its surface and help in its defense. This microscopic army works 24/7 to fight off any foreign invaders, without which, our immune system would be overwhelmed in short order, and we would die.

YOUR RESIDENT BACTERIA OR MICROBIOME

Most people are totally unaware of the role of beneficial (good) bacteria that live all over the surface as well as the inside of our bodies, especially in our intestines.

The vast majority of the bacteria covering our skin and mucous membranes are of five types. Some specialize in defending the valleys like hair follicles and deep pores, others swarm the surface looking for a fight.

These bacteria occupy an area and act as a local army, defending their turf to the death. If an invading bacterium tries to occupy an area of your skin or your intestines, it must kick the ass of the locals or it's a no go. The good flora or bacteria are literally fighting for their lives and that of their entire colony. If they lose, the disease-causing bacteria will replace them, and thus you become infected.

Thus the great push for people to use probiotics (and prebiotics to feed them properly) supplements to continue to send reinforcements to your good intestinal flora.

These good resident florae are killed by antibiotics that are too frequently overprescribed to Americans. The situation is even worse in foreign countries, where frequently, patients do not even need a prescription. They merely show up at a pharmacy and ask for penicillin or whatever antibiotic they might have heard of in the past. This leads to horrific overuse of antibiotics and the creation of resistance.

Resistance occurs from overuse of antibiotics by selecting out for bugs that are not killed by the initial round of antibiotics and/or the recurrent use of antibiotics in the same patient. Patients inadvertently cause this by stopping their antibiotics when they feel better. They think they are cured, so why continue?

As doctors, we prescribe antibiotics for a specific period of time, say for example, ten days. The first few days, the least resistant bacteria are killed; over the course of the ten days, the more resistant ones are killed. Now, if you stop after six days because you are asymptomatic (no symptoms), you are leaving the more resistant bacteria; and unopposed, they rapidly multiply.

Another mechanism for the development of bacterial (and fungal) resistance is by mutations in their DNA. The new mutated bacteria have developed a gene that confers resistance. Sometimes, this gene is transmitted between bacteria spreading resistance to other bacteria.

Another source of resistance are large factory farms that we have in the United States. These farms that raise pigs, chickens, cows, turkeys, and other animals are the primary users of antibiotics in the United States. They account for approximately 70 percent of our antibiotic use.

The runoff from these farms is rich with mutated bacterial species (and viruses) that are resistant to the multiple antibiotics used on these farms. These super resistant bacteria are known as *superbugs*. These infections are devastating to humans since we use many of the same antibiotics as the farms. It is estimated that over seven hundred thousand people die annually worldwide from infections from these mutated superbugs.

On a smaller scale, the same thing happens in patients who recurrently use antibiotics. Eventually, they don't work as effectively, and hence they require stronger and stronger antibiotics or combinations of them. You should always try to be as prudent as possible in your use of antibiotics for that reason and also for its devastating effect upon your body's own microbiome or population of good bacteria.

Our bodies were not designed to have our gut flora and other populations of good/beneficial bacteria periodically eradicated. We have no evolutionary mechanism to replace these bacterial colonies, many of whom were given to us by our mothers.

Keep in mind the unbelievable reproductive capacity of bacteria. The bacteria that inhabit our body, as in the intestines for example, have an average life span of about twenty minutes. Ponder that for a moment... That means in one day, seventy-two generations of bacteria will have evolved. In human years, seventy-two generations would bring us back before Christ.

Knowing that, you can imagine what happens when we are infected with a bacterium for ten days, for example. That would cover the life span of 720 generations of bacteria, giving them ample time to mutate to try to evade our bodies' defenses. That is why drug resistance developed. Now, multidrug resistant species of bacteria are emerging, making treatment with even combinations of antibiotics useless.

Now, you can understand why the focus of my medical practice and this book is to help you build your own "wall of immunity" in order to prevent infections rather than worry about treating multidrug resistant mutations.

It is interesting to note that when you compare the microbiome of patients in the Western world to those of indigenous tribes from the Amazon or Africa, we have a fraction of the good bacteria in our bodies, and with considerably less diversity as well.

Sometimes we absolutely need a course of antibiotics. After such a course, you should spend the next few weeks taking probiotic bacteria, eating fermented foods and prodigious amounts of prebiotic foods to feed your new friends. This has no downside and will help to at least partially repopulate your gut.

Your gut microbiome helps to digest food, thus releasing energy and also produces vitamins. They produce mostly B vitamins such as biotin, folate, thiamine, niacin, and B12.

The number of bacterial cells in our microbiome is astonishing. Currently, it is estimated they compose about ten times the number of cells in our entire body! As our understanding of how the microbiome functions evolves, it is becoming quite evident that they shape everything from our weight to our immunity and very likely even to our evolution. I think the more we learn the more it blurs the line between how we think of ourselves as humans and our microbiome, the separation rapidly disappears.

As I have just shown you, your skin acts as an impenetrable wall, along with its secreted oils, macrophages, and beneficial microbes, that is quite formidable. Let's take a look at how other body organs defend themselves.

YOUR RESPIRATORY SYSTEM

Air entering our body provides oxygen for energy and life and carries out exhaled waste or carbon dioxide that is deadly if retained.

The part of the respiratory system that transports air to our alveoli or air sacs is called the conducting zone. The place where gases are exchanged is known as the respiratory zone.

In the conducting zone, oxygen-rich air must enter either through our nose or mouth and proceed down the trachea, where it branches off to either your right or left bronchus to their respective lungs.

After each bronchus, the air travels through progressively smaller bronchioles until it reaches the alveolar duct, through which it travels to the alveoli or air sacs. This is where your body interfaces with the outer world by taking in air and soaking up its oxygen while ridding itself of its carbon dioxide. This is vital for your survival. However, at the same time, this is where we are really vulnerable to airborne toxins, pollution, particulate matter, and of course germs of all types, including the current bad boy of viruses, COVID-19.

Your entire respiratory tract from your nose and sinuses to the ducts to your alveoli are all lined with cells that have cilia covering their surfaces. These cilia are tiny hairlike projections that vibrate in unison. The cilia cover your airways and in turn are covered by a layer of mucus. This mucus layer is full of substances that kill and remove invading germs.

The mucus does this by enzymes called lysozymes that destroy bacterial invaders. The cilia beat in a rhythmic fashion towards your mouth, thus passing bacteria-laden mucus along like a person being carried above the heads of the crowd in a mosh pit. These cilia are destroyed by smoking, thus making smokers susceptible to lung infections, such as bronchitis and pneumonia.

Once the cilia are destroyed, the goblet cells continue to produce mucus just like before; but now, this mucus pools in the lungs since without the cilia, there is no mechanism for its removal. Consequently, in those smokers, they develop a hacking cough, which is their bodies' attempt to expectorate or cough up the mucus. Hence the classic smokers' cough that many chronic smokers have.

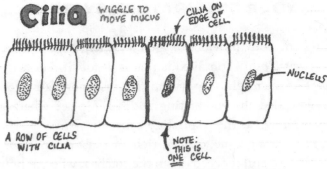

Courtesy of not Rocket science

In your lungs, there are air sacs known as alveoli. They look like clusters of grapes on a grapevine, which is your airways. The alveoli are where the respiratory zone is. This is where the action is in our lungs.

To help further protect our bodies, these air sacs or alveoli are also lined with macrophages that gobble up dust particles and invading germs.

Our lungs also have a mechanism that triggers a cough reflex when there is an accumulation of mucus on top of the cilia that needs to be mechanically cleared. Coughing results from an irritation of our airways. It can also be the result of stimulation of receptors in the ear, lung, diaphragm, and even the stomach.

You might have noticed that sometimes when you are wiggling a Q-tip around inside your ear, it makes you cough. That is from stimulation of the cough reflex. It is a very powerful way by which your body is able to send a rush of air from your lungs through your airways to your mouth.

You can imagine, from the perspective of the surface of your airways, this is like cyclone-force winds passing overhead, carrying along globs of infected mucus from the cilia along with foreign particles such as dust, smoke particles, and other toxins. Coughing is a very effective way to clear your lungs.

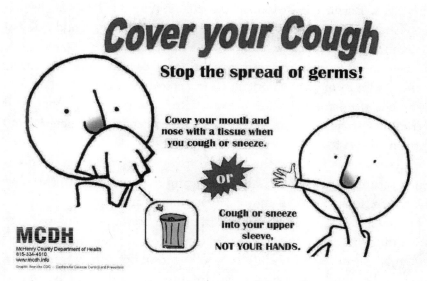

Another way your respiratory tract clears infections is when your nose, sinuses, and nasal passages are infected, they will pour out fluid to mechanically flush their surface, thus giving you what is medically known as rhinitis or a runny nose. It will also do that when exposed to allergens such as pollen and dust. That is allergic rhinitis, hence mechanically washing the offending allergens away by flooding the surface of your nose with fluid.

EYES

Our eyes tear when exposed to an irritant or an allergen, helping the body mechanically flush our eyes and eliminate the problem. Both tears and mucus contain enzymes called lysozymes that dissolve the bacterial cell wall, killing them.

These enzymes work well to kill any bacteria or fungus that might be attacking the surface of your eyes. Tears mechanically flush your eyes while at the same time disinfecting and lubricating them.

EARS

By now, surely you have noticed that every opening into the body is protected by various means. Your ears do so by producing cerumen or earwax. Earwax comes in various colors, with the Japanese having the weirdest color of gray. That is one of those millions of odd tidbits I remember from medical school.

No one is quite sure of the function of earwax. We can surely surmise a lot from its components. Earwax is mostly composed of dead skin cells from the ear canal mixed with a potpourri of other stuff including lysozyme—that you already learned is both antibacterial and antifungal.

Lysozyme is used by the body in many of its secretions, such as blood serum, gastric juices, saliva, breast milk, earwax, and respiratory tract secretions. You can figure out its importance for protecting an infant by its amazing concentration in human breast milk compared to cow milk.

In breast milk, it is 1,600 to 3,000 times more concentrated than cow's milk, thus conferring to an infant a huge dose of lysosomal enzymes. These lysozymes will destroy any bacteria or fungi in its path, thus protecting the infant until it is able to develop its own immune system. Hence one of many reasons for the importance of breastfeeding your children.

THE GI TRACT

The GI tract starts with the oral cavity and the solution of enzymes and antibodies in its saliva. Saliva is replete with enzymes, white blood cells (immune cells), and antimicrobial immunoglobulins. This is the body's first line of defense once you enter the mouth. That area is also full of lymphatics acting as a second line of defense.

Tonsils are patches of lymphatics acting as sentinels guarding the nose, mouth, and throat. In the very back of the nasal cavity lie the adenoids that protects you from pathogens coming into the nose before it reaches the oral pharynx.

In the oral cavity lie three other sets of tonsils on the palate and under the tongue. In addition to which there are lymphatic networks, both superficially and in deep tissues of the neck. More on lymphatics in a little bit.

Other mechanisms that your GI tract uses if it is under attack are nausea, vomiting, and diarrhea. It tries to expel the invaders by ejecting them out of your mouth or by shortening the time they are in contact with your intestines by pouring out fluid that gives you diarrhea and flushing the pathogens out of your colon. For that reason, taking medication to stop a new or acute case of diarrhea is oftentimes self-defeating and can be dangerous. Since you are now absorbing toxins, you should be expelling.

Another formidable line of defense is your stomach. Any germs that were able to pass the enzymes and antibodies of the mouth and the lymphatic system now travel down your esophagus into the acid pit of your stomach. Invading bacteria also get trapped in the mucus of the GI tract and are swallowed and then travel down the esophagus into the stomach where they are killed and dissolved by its acid.

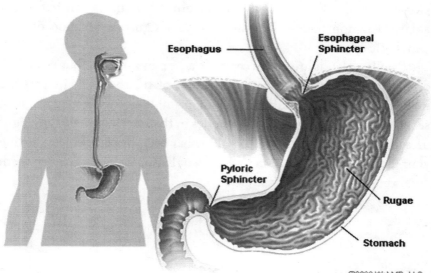

©2009 WebMD, LLC.

Stomach acid is not a mild acid; it has a pH around 2, which is an extraordinarily strong acid, akin to battery acid. Most microorganisms (germs) are not able to survive this pH and thus the low number of infections of the lower GI tract that do not involve breaking down the mucosal barrier. This is quite a formidable defensive barrier for our immune system.

The acid in the stomach is made of potassium chloride, sodium chloride, and hydrochloric acid, and there are also digestive enzymes such as pepsin. You can see the importance of chloride; we will get to this later when I discuss using magnesium chloride.

THE LYMPHATIC SYSTEM

The lymphatic system is cool. It is a hybrid of the circulatory and immune systems. It drains lymph that circulates through all the tissues of the body; thus it is delivering samples from each area to one of your body's six hundred lymph nodes.

Lymph nodes are little forts that process these lymphatic tissue samples, and if it finds any antigens or foreign proteins that it does not recognize, it attacks them. This results in the lymph node swelling. If it is near the surface as in your neck, you will have what is known as swollen glands. These swollen glands are not glands at all but rather enlarged lymph nodes. They are always a sign of activation of your lymphatic system.

Swollen glands are not necessarily a sign of infection but rather are often enlarged simply from presentation of microorganisms that are eventually inactivated/killed. A good example of that is many times I see patients with enlarged lymph nodes in their neck, without any signs or symptoms of infection. This often happens from briskly brushing your teeth, which sends bacteria into your lymphatics, resulting in them enlarging to meet the threat.

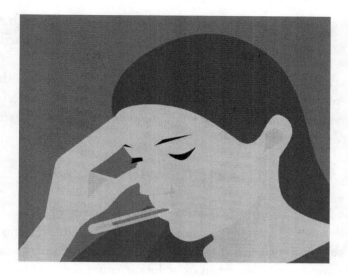

FEVER

Once these mechanisms fail, your body takes out its "ace in the hole" fever. Our bodies can only become infected by bacteria or viruses, or any pathogen for that matter, that live at or close to our body temperature: 98.6 degrees F. It is a very narrow range—too low they die, too high they die.

Remember this: your body does nothing by random. Fever is not accidental. Your body is raising its own temperature in a race to kill off the bacteria before it harms itself. If a fever goes too high in a last-ditch effort to kill the invaders, you could have seizures and even death.

So, what do people foolishly do? They take aspirin, acetaminophen (Tylenol), ibuprofen (Motrin or Advil), naproxen (Naprosyn or Aleve) all in a futile, foolish attempt to lower their temperatures. The only thing taking any of these antipyretics (fever-reducing medications) does is block your body's greatest line of defense and prolong your illness by literally working against your own immunity.

The only time you should take a fever-reducing medication is if your temperature is going above 102 degrees F, and only then if you absolutely must due to discomfort or delirium.

In addition to which, aspirin should never be given to children since it may cause Reye's syndrome. This includes children and teenagers up to the age of fifteen. Reye's syndrome damages the liver, which releases ammonia into the blood, which crosses the blood-brain barrier and damages the brain.

Once again, you can see the repeating pattern: once the skin barrier, respiratory, gastrointestinal (GI) tract, or local bacterial flora is overcome, the only backup is your body's immune system. And what an incredible second line of defense it is.

YOUR AMAZING IMMUNE SYSTEM

Your body's most primitive form of immunity is called its innate immunity. This is what you are born with as your first immune system and is genetically determined. It is distinguished from the adaptive immune system, which evolves or adapts as you grow.

The innate immune system works by sounding the alarm about an invader of some kind. The invader may be bacterial, parasitic, viral, or even a protein it does not recognize as self. It does so by releasing chemical mediators called cytokines, which in turn attract or recruit other immune cells.

This innate immunity works by a series of complex proteins found in the blood, such as the complement system and interleukin 1 and interferon. It jumps into action immediately upon recognition of nonself or foreign substances.

The complement system is a series of proteins that swim through your blood looking for trouble. As they swim through the blood, they are surrounded by a sea of antibodies, each of which is looking for one specific antigen, be they foreign proteins or microorganisms or infectious agents.

The antibodies bind with the specific antigen they have been waiting for. This activates complement proteins swimming by. The complement proteins are the "hit men" that destroy these agents and further activate the immune system. They are called complement because they "complement" the function of antibodies.

Interleukin-1 is responsible for producing fever, thus highlighting its importance in the body's defense. It also causes the release of acute phase proteins from the liver, which charge up the immune system and lead to inflammation.

Interferon is a family of immune regulating proteins. Its job is to protect certain cells that have adjacent cells exposed to bacteria and/or viral infections, parasites, and other antigens. Its most important function occurs when it is secreted in response to a viral infection. Interferon causes adjacent noninfected cells to produce proteins that interfere (thus its name) with the virus, infecting those healthy cells. Another example of the body's ingenious defense mechanism.

The next line of immunity is called passive immunity, since these antibodies to foreign antigens are made outside the body by the mother. These antibodies are passed to the fetus and protect the newborn infant for about the first six to twelve months. After that time, the infant's immune system must take over and become responsible for its own immunity.

Most of these antibodies are passed via the placenta to the fetus during the last three months of pregnancy. The types of antibodies passed from the mother depend upon the mother's exposure to various infections. If she has had mumps or measles, then those antibodies will be present and passed along. Antibodies are also passed to the fetus via breastfeeding.

The first few days of breastfeeding contain a different thick yellow breast milk known as colostrum. This is particularly rich in antibodies and gives another strong blast of antibodies to help the infant. Children who are born premature or who are not breastfed do not have this advantage of the transfer of huge amounts of antibodies and therefore have immune systems that are inherently weaker. Hence the importance of breast feeding.

This next line of immunity is called acquired immunity or sometimes the adaptive immune system. This involves cellular immunity, primarily from white cells circulating in the blood.

These white blood cells, or leukocytes, circulate in the blood and perform constant immune surveillance, looking for invading bacteria, viruses or parasites, and damaged cells. It does this by looking at the proteins on their surface, where it is able to tell the difference between your body's cells or self and foreign cells or proteins or nonself.

These cells then compare the protein they found to the library of proteins that they have already made antibodies to from prior exposure. If there is a match, they then churn out large numbers of antibodies to attack these germs, or anti-venom to attack venom, and anti-toxins to neutralize toxins.

You should note that having anti-venom and anti-toxin antibodies is not natural but rather comes from previous exposure to venom or toxins.

If there is no match between the new protein antigen and the library of antigens possessed by the white blood cells, then they begin to produce novel antibodies from scratch to kill or neutralize the new invader.

White cells are stored in the thymus, spleen, bone marrow, and lymph nodes. They come in two main types: phagocytes and lymphocytes.

Phagocytes ingest or eat foreign germs and proteins and thereby inactivate them. They come in four types; the most numerous by far are the neutrophils followed by monocytes, macrophages, and mast cells.

The lymphocytes are where the memory of previous infections is stored. They are made in the bone marrow and are called B cells or B lymphocytes. Some migrate to the thymus gland and are called T cells or T lymphocytes.

The job of the B cells is to produce antibodies and to release substances that attract its big brother, the T cells. The B cells produce antibodies that act as missiles, attacking the specific invader it had matched to from its memory.

The T cells destroy the invading organisms and send out a distress call to attract other white cells from the phagocyte lineage to help them devour the invading microorganisms (germs).

This chapter has illustrated for you the various ingenious systems our body uses to defend itself. As you have hopefully learned, it is a very elaborate, complex system, with redundant backups and a long memory. It serves our bodies 24/7, preventing infections of all types until it is overwhelmed, and we become infected.

Remember, the only way you can catch any infection is by the infection defeating your many layers of immunity. Hence the importance of boosting your immunity, to "raise the bar" or "build the wall" that the invader must overcome. All the various components of the body's amazing immune system are all just cinder blocks in that wall that work together in amazing harmony twenty-four hours a day, seven days a week.

In my opinion, it is preferable to routinely boost your immunity by ways that I will teach you, then to try to conquer an infection that has already invaded your body.

First of all, any infection is damaging the body part it is infecting. Treating an infection almost always causes collateral damage either to vital organs or to our wonderful microbiome, neither of which is good for us. Hence the old saying from Benjamin Franklin, "An ounce of prevention is worth a pound of cure."

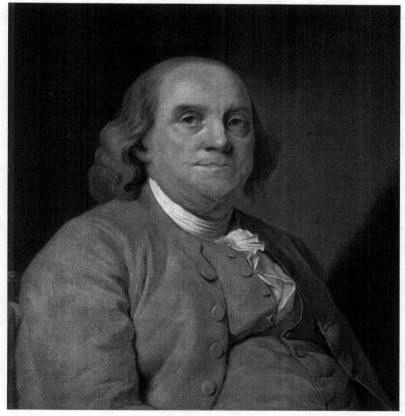

You have to love Benjamin Franklin—what a cool guy. He was a scientist, inventor, author, businessman, diplomat, and quite a rogue in his day, even with that body!

CHAPTER THREE

WHAT ARE YOUR SYMPTOMS?

Colds, flu, and coronaviruses all have similar symptoms because they all start by infecting the upper and lower respiratory tract. That fact is the reason why it is so difficult for doctors to discern one from the other.

One possible hint as to what is infecting you is the time of year. There is definitely a flu season (see the chart below). Much to the astonishment of the public, the typical flu season has some coronaviruses as well, as many as 15 percent! That actually might turn out to be a good thing, since for those people, it might confer at least partial immunity to COVID-19. The jury is still out on that, but in my opinion, it sounds plausible since it works that way with other families of viruses.

That certainly was the case with the Spanish flu of 1918. During that pandemic, it primarily killed young adults and spared those who were middle-aged and very young. The sparing of the young was due to other reasons. However, the middle-aged and older were apparently infected with a flu that was close enough in its genetic makeup to the Spanish flu that they had antibodies that protected them.

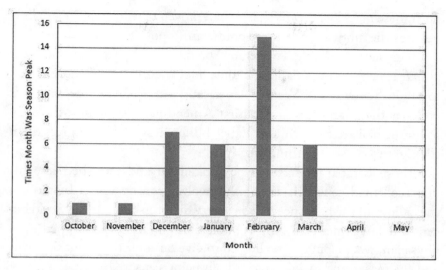

As you can plainly see, the four-month period from December to March is flu season. If you have symptoms you think are the flu and it is May through September, it is highly unlikely to be the flu. Although the dates I am citing are in the Northern Hemisphere. The flu season is the polar opposite of that in the Southern Hemisphere (no pun intended), and it is all year around at the equator. I will explain more about that when I discuss vitamin D's role.

COVID-19 so far has not run the usual course of a seasonal respiratory tract infection. It is difficult to determine if that is partially or in whole due to our response to it. Never before in history have we had a "reverse quarantine." By that, I mean quarantining the entire population rather than the sick or the super vulnerable like the elderly. In addition to which this insane lockdown has prevented the normal spread of a virus through the population.

Clearly, now that we have a year's experience with this virus (at the time of this writing), it appears that masks, quarantines, and lockdowns have done nothing, in my opinion, but delay the developing of herd immunity and, in effect, has prolonged and vastly amplified the effect of a virus that now has the same death rate as the seasonal flu!

In my opinion, it makes absolutely no sense; and as our collective experience with COVID-19 increases, it is becoming very obvious that countries like Sweden that did not quarantine have the same infection rates as those that did. So that begs the question, why do we continue to push these mass lockdowns that are not proven to work at all? Dare I say perhaps the motivation of these politicians is political and not medical?

I am sure Facebook, Twitter, or YouTube would flag that statement as hate speech and an unallowed conspiracy theory. All the more reason to say it. Screw them! We are Americans and are born free, and that includes the guarantees of the First Amendment, freedom of speech. Who the hell are these Silicon Valley billionaires, and what gives them the right to censor anything we say?

Those companies have to be broken up and punished for this unprecedented censoring that only involves conservatives. Incredibly, they allow all the hate speech from petty dictators around the world but censor fellow Americans. This is intolerable and has to be stopped. As a physician, we no longer are allowed to give our opinion about the virus and the masks and lockdowns without being censored.

Medicine thrives on different opinions and theories that compete in the marketplace of ideas; if your opinion can be disproven by another, then so be it. Without this exchange, all we have is medical dogma, and that is very dangerous. We need to be able to express our opinions and let the best ideas win!

COVID-19 is not evolving as it spreads through the population. It is not acting as a natural virus would, leading to the question, is it man-made? There have been some Chinese scientists that have come forward and said just that, but the mainstream media's complete lack of interest in pursuing this is utterly amazing, and at the same time quite disheartening.

On the other hand, it is mutating as all viruses do after passing through millions of human hosts. As I mentioned earlier, it already has twenty-three known mutations, and that number will surely go up even further. Viruses almost exclusively mutate to lesser lethality as the virus tries to eventually coexist with the host.

Our DNA is proof of this since it is loaded with viral DNA from centuries past. The most recent estimates are that 8 percent of human DNA is actually from viruses, most often retroviruses from millions of years ago! And you were worried about mixing your DNA with that loser first husband of yours!

As we gain more experience with COVID-19, we are coming to the realization that it is not acting at all like other corona viruses. It appears to be striking different organs in each patient, with no discernable pattern. Our understanding of how COVID-19 affects patients is in constant evolution as we gain more experience.

As these various viruses enter the upper respiratory tract, they infect the nose, sinuses, ears, and throat.

The ears get infected via the eustachian tubes, which connect the nasal pharynx with the ear, thus providing a path for invading germs.

This is the area where most folks get their first symptoms of a respiratory infection of any kind. You develop a runny nose (rhinitis), sinus obstruction with that pressure like sensation in your forehead and behind your eyes, often accompanied by a sinus headache. You will know it is a sinus headache when you bend over, it will cause a sudden increase in pressure in your head. You feel like your head is going to explode.

Your hearing may be affected by fluid in your middle ear, which will also cause balance problems and even vertigo (dizziness). Often, your ears will "pop" as the pressures change in the middle ear and your eustachian tube opens from its usual collapsed state. You may even develop an earache (otalgia) from the pressure buildup. You can force your eustachian tubes open by breathing out forcibly, with your nose and mouth closed. You can do this several times repeatedly. "Tooting" your nose like this will sometimes help open a blocked eustachian tube. Medically, that is known as a Valsalva maneuver.

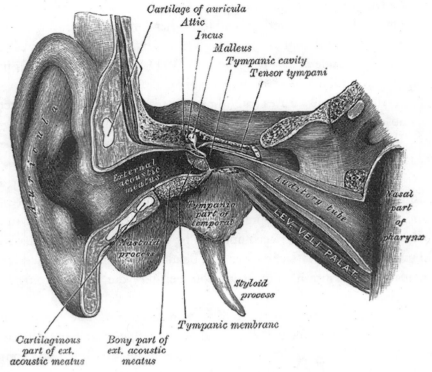

Eustachian tube (labelled as auditory tube)
Courtesy of Gray's Anatomy

The usual symptoms of COVID-19 infection begin when it travels to the lower respiratory tract or lungs. Those symptoms are fever, cough, and shortness of breath. The shortness of breath becomes severe as the infection progresses. Ultimately, most patients present to the hospital with problems breathing.

Sooner or later, many eventually go into respiratory failure, and many succumb due to ARDS (acute respiratory distress syndrome) and bacterial pneumonias. ARDS means that your air sacs or alveoli in your lungs are filled with fluid, causing the lung to be quite stiff and unable to allow proper oxygen absorption.

This rapid progression of symptoms from hospitalization to respiratory failure and ultimately intubation is what was overwhelming the hospital ICU (intensive care unit) beds, by utilizing all their ventilators. In addition to which, coronavirus patients seem to linger quite a long time before either recuperating or dying. This ties up hospital beds, especially in the ICU.

One of the major problems with controlling the COVID-19 pandemic is the fact that the vast majority of patients either have no symptoms or just feel a little under the weather as if they had caught a mild cold.

Since they are asymptomatic (have no symptoms), they are out and about doing their normal activities, unaware that they are shedding infectious virus particles onto objects where they can remain for days, and to other people. There is currently some controversy as to whether these asymptomatic patients are shedding virus and are thus infective to others or not.

This ever-increasing pool of asymptomatic (they have no symptoms) or mild to moderately symptomatic (feeling like they have a cold or a mild flu) patients has caused the death rate to drop to levels comparable with the flu.

When we were first testing, we only could test people who came to the hospital and were sick, thus the percentage of those patients who died became our death rate. Now, since we have been mass testing for many months, the asymptomatic pool is ever expanding, which is good news. That in turn has caused a progressive drop in the death rate from COVID-19.

There are also two other problems contributing to skewered numbers of COVID-19 deaths. If you have COVID-19 and you are hit by a car, that counts as a COVID death.

I had a patient who was about 400 lbs., uncontrolled diabetic with a heart condition. She unfortunately dropped dead, and her funeral home wanted me to write COVID-19 as her cause of death. I of course did not, and when has it become appropriate for a funeral home to request a cause of death from a physician? Year 2020 kept getting weirder and weirder.

The second problem, are the tests reliable? Elon Musk just announced that he took four COVID-19 tests simultaneously, same nurse, lab, and equipment. Two came out positive and two negative. That does not exactly instill confidence in anyone. It is very much like voting in the

2020 presidential elections, not exactly a testimonial to election fairness! However, I digress.

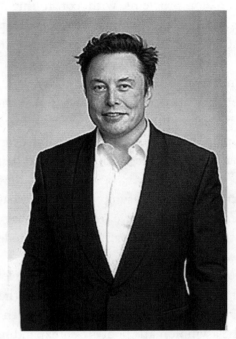

Lately, with coronavirus, two new symptoms have emerged, anosmia or loss of the sense of smell, and either markedly decreased sense of taste or hypogeusia, or even total absence of taste or ageusia. These two symptoms were never associated with colds, flus, and even coronaviruses.

They are rapidly becoming very important symptoms of COVID-19 infection. Especially in light of the fact that these symptoms are quite unusual and not something most primary care doctors frequently encounter. That also highlights where COVID-19 is entering our bodies—through our nasal passages and mouth.

It has become increasingly apparent to the medical world that COVID-19 is not like previous viruses from the coronavirus family. They almost exclusively infected the respiratory system. We are now seeing COVID-19 infecting every organ in the body. Now, that being said, the overwhelming majority of cases still involve the respiratory system.

Other less common symptoms that are infrequent but are increasing in numbers, as the overall number of cases rises, are headache, confusion, mental status changes, and even seizures in some cases. Another increasingly common symptom is diarrhea.

COVID-19 has been isolated from respiratory secretions, blood, and feces so far, and all these are naturally infective.

As this COVID-19 pandemic evolves, doctors are noting different symptoms. Recently, discoloration of toes has been named COVID toes and is now being included as an unusual presentation of the virus. It is now known to involve not just toes but fingers as well.

We are now learning this is due to inflammation of the blood vessels or vasculitis. It now appears that the viral spike proteins are able to attach and infect the endothelial cells that line our blood vessels and appear to be able to also cross the blood-brain barrier and enter the brain.

Vasculitis is proving to be a quite common and increasingly severe complication of COVID-19. Vasculitis is the medical term that means inflammation of the circulatory or vascular system. The vascular system has three parts: the arterial system, which includes arteries and their smaller arterioles, the venous system with veins and their smaller venules, and capillaries, which connect the arterioles and the venules.

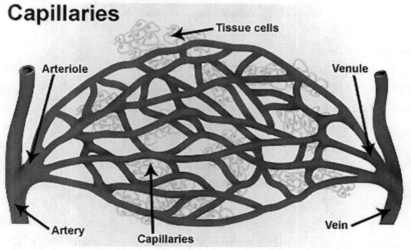

Drawing courtesy of the National Institute of Health
and the National Cancer Institute

We now know that COVID-19 infects all organs and the entire circulatory system. When it infects the endothelial cells, it leads to inflammation of the blood vessels or vasculitis. The infected endothelial cells trigger an extreme immune response. This infection and the resulting inflammation leads to thrombosis or clotting of the blood vessels.

These clots block the blood flow, and this in turn leads to damage of the tissues "downstream." It most often affects the hands and feet but can strike anywhere, including the brain and the heart.

What do these vasculitis lesions look and feel like you ponder? Typically, these are reddened areas of your fingers or toes, but can be on other areas of skin. They may be mildly itchy, tender, and sometimes lead to blisters.

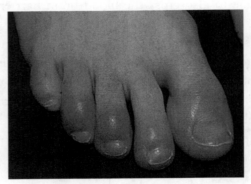

Photo courtesy of Wikipedia

Another recently recognized symptom is pink eye and swollen eyes. Pink eye is known medically as conjunctivitis, and as the name so aptly implies, it causes the white of the eye to appear pink in color.

Colds and flus have remarkably similar symptoms to coronavirus infections. There are, however, some notable exceptions: the flu usually causes a severe headache (made worse by coughing), severe myalgias (muscle pain), and extreme fatigue.

Colds usually just are a much milder version of the flu without the muscle aches and just a mild headache. Very rarely do either cause shortness of breath to the degree we are currently seeing with COVID-19. Nor do colds and flu cause other symptoms that COVID-19 does, such as diarrhea, conjunctivitis, vasculitis, and loss of the sense of taste and/ or smell.

Symptoms of various respiratory tract infections usually point directly to the area involved. If you have a frontal headache, meaning pressure behind your eyes or in your forehead area, you are most likely dealing with a frontal sinus infection. There may or not be rhinitis or a runny nose with that. Once the nose starts running, it usually helps relieve the pressure in the forehead that is causing the sinus headache.

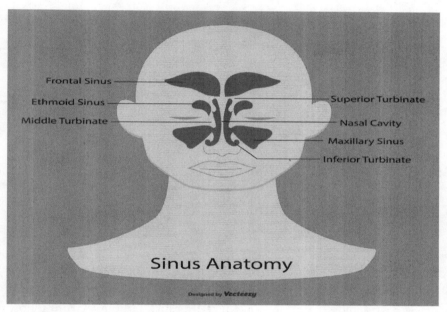

Sinus Anatomy

Frontal Sinus
Ethmoid Sinus
Middle Turbinate
Superior Turbinate
Nasal Cavity
Maxillary Sinus
Inferior Turbinate

Designed by **Vecteezy**

If your upper teeth hurt, this is also a sign of a sinus infection—not your frontal sinuses but rather your maxillary sinuses. Many a patient has gone to the dentist thinking for sure they had a bad tooth and was pleasantly surprised to find out it was a maxillary sinus infection instead. No one likes that high-pitched whistle of that dental drill. My good friend and dentist Mark Longobardi openly mocks me for being such a wimp in his dental chair as I squirm and sweat. I am guilty as charged.

The reason your upper teeth hurt with a maxillary sinus infection is that their nerve roots run adjacent to the sinuses; when they swell, they put pressure on those nerves, leading to a toothache. It usually involves the upper rear molars. You can differentiate it from a toothache since it typically involves several teeth.

Coronavirus vs Cold vs FLU vs Allergies

SYMPTOMS	COVID-19*	COLD	FLU	ALLERGIES
Fever	Common (100 F or higher)	Rare	High (100-102F, can last 3-4 days)	No
Headache	Sometimes	Rare	Intense	Sometimes
General aches, pains	Sometimes	Slight	Common (often severe)	No
Fatigue, weakness	Sometimes	Slight	Common (often severe)	Sometimes
Extreme exhaustion	Sometimes (progresses slowly)	Never	Common (starts early)	No
Stuffy nose	Rare	Common	Sometimes	Common
Sneezing	Rare	Common	Sometimes	Common
Sore throat	Rare	Common	Common	No
Cough	Common	Mild to moderate	Common (can become severe)	Sometimes
Shortness of breath	In more serious infections	Rare	Rare	Common
Runny nose	Rare	Common	Sometimes	Common
Diarrhea	Sometimes	No	Sometimes**	No

*Information is still evolving **Sometimes for children

Allergies also are often confused with infections, but allergies do not cause fever, myalgias (muscle aches), purulent sputum (green or other nasty colors), and does not usually cause fatigue. A runny nose from allergies will be clear in color.

Allergies are often seasonal in nature, striking in the spring when all the trees, bushes, and flowers are sending streams of pollen into the air, with a second peak in the fall. Allergies usually cause sneezing, itchy eyes, runny nose, and sometimes wheezing but not usually a cough. Allergies often cause an itchy sensation in the nose and/or throat.

Symptoms of a sore throat are pretty straightforward—your throat hurts, and it might burn as you swallow food or beverages. You might also have swollen glands or lymph nodes in your neck. If you still have your tonsils, you might have tonsillitis, in which case at the base of your tongue on either side, you will see a marble-sized swelling—those are your tonsils. Usually, swallowing becomes not only painful but mechanically difficult. Sometimes, you will see yellow spots on your tonsils—this is a further sign of infection and is caused by pus pockets in your tonsils.

If your larynx or voice box is involved, you will most likely become hoarse, with a raspy voice that makes you sound like former President Bill Clinton.

Earaches are also due primarily to ear infections. Sometimes, it is eustachian tube dysfunction with pressure buildup in your middle ear. The middle ear is normally a closed space filled with air; it can only equalize with the outside world by your eustachian tube opening and relieving some of that buildup of air pressure. If your eustachian tube is not opening and closing properly, this is known as eustachian tube dysfunction and will lead to ear pain.

Infections involving your nasal passages will usually result in rhinitis or runny nose, as your body attempts to wash away any irritant or infectious agent. If your nasal discharge (snot) is clear, that usually indicates a viral infection. If it turns green, it is indicative of a bacterial infection. That is an important distinction because only bacterial infections will respond to antibiotics.

A lower respiratory tract infection is one that involves areas below your larynx or voice box. It primarily is an infection of your bronchi (your airways leading to your lungs) and lungs. An infection of your bronchial airways is known as bronchitis. If it spreads into your lung tissue, it is known as pneumonia. Bronchitis frequently precedes pneumonia, but not always.

Pneumonia is much more serious than bronchitis. Both conditions involve bouts of coughing, with or without production of sputum (phlegm). Once again, the color of sputum is very important. White or clear sputum is typically from a viral infection, whereas green or brown sputum is typically bacterial in origin.

In pneumonia, sputum is sometimes mixed with blood or actually tinted by blood into a rusty-looking appearance. That is never a good sign. Pneumonia is typically associated with dyspnea or shortness of breath since it involves the alveoli where oxygen is absorbed. Fluid- and pus-filled alveoli will not have the surface area they need for adequate oxygen absorption, and hence blood oxygen levels will drop, resulting in shortness of breath. Pneumonia is typically life threatening in the elderly, who often succumb to it.

Other symptoms of pneumonia are rapid shallow breathing (a normal respiratory rate varies between individuals and is usually about 18, but can range from 12 to 20 breaths per minute) and labored breathing, sometimes using accessory muscles of their abdomen to help move their diaphragm. If severe, the patient may develop a dusky, blue-tinged appearance.

These are not good signs and are indicative or current or pending respiratory failure. Respiratory failure is a medical emergency, and if you have any of those symptoms, you should report to your local hospital immediately.

Patients oftentimes have loud wheezing as well, which is a whistling sound as they inspire or breath in. They oftentimes will also have severe bouts of coughing that come in spurts as the body attempts to blow out or clear its airways that are becoming progressively clogged with mucus/pus and sometimes blood mixture.

You can easily discern an upper respiratory tract infection from a more serious lower respiratory tract infection. Upper respiratory tract infections will involve a runny nose, sneezing, headache, and sore throat. Whereas symptoms of a lower respiratory tract infection will primarily be coughing, fatigue (often severe), shortness of breath, and perhaps a bluish discoloration to a patient's skin—and typically, the patient is much sicker upon presentation.

That basically concludes our tour of the respiratory tract and the symptoms of infection of each of its components.

CHAPTER FOUR

NUTRITIONAL DEFICIENCIES AND YOUR IMMUNITY

This includes colds, sinus infections, sore throats, flu, bronchitis, pneumonia, and COVID-19.

In this chapter, I will provide you with several basic things you can do to prevent infections with personal hygiene and also ways to boost your immune system and help prevent colds, flu, and COVID-19. Many of the methods I am touching upon in this chapter will be covered much more deeply in following chapters. This is more of an introduction to cleansing and toughening your body and preventing infections.

All the methods I am going to describe below to prevent and treat coronaviruses, colds, and flu are no guarantee. They are merely your best bet at preventing and, if you do get it, of having the mildest course of infection.

The reason I say that is that there are many other factors that contribute to your immune function, many adversely. Lack of sleep, stress, depression, drug or alcohol use, comorbidities (having other medical conditions) such as diabetes, hypertension, COPD, HIV, cancers of any type—all put the kibosh on your health.

PERSONAL HYGIENE: KING OF PREVENTION

One of the biggest factors that will determine if you catch any respiratory tract infection is good personal hygiene. Handwashing is king, there is no doubt about it.

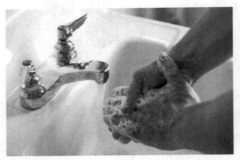

WHY SOAP AND WATER ARE SO EFFECTIVE

Basic hygiene is and always will be the king of infectious disease prevention. Respiratory tract infections such as colds, flus, and coronaviruses all must find their way to your nose or mouth to enter your body.

Touching your face with hands that are covered with live virus is a sure way to catch a respiratory virus (along with someone coughing directly into your face). Let's face it, it is shocking how often we touch our faces. We do it a hell of a lot—in fact, almost constantly. There is a good chance your hands are touching some part of your face right now. For that reason, when it comes to prevention, handwashing is king!

Soap works its wonders due to its chemical structure. Chemically, soap is known as an amphiphile. This means that it has one end that is attracted to water, and its opposite end is attracted to fats or oils.

Viral particles like coronavirus are enveloped in a fat or lipid coating, the soap tears this apart, killing the virus. Soap also breaks the attachment of viruses to oils in your skin, mechanically washing them off your skin. That one-two punch allows soap to kill and/or flush away viruses and other germs effectively and inexpensively, without harmful side effects.

Hand sanitizers work because they are over 60 percent alcohol, which kills germs on contact.

Remember the old cowboy pictures when they would make a guy drink a lot of alcohol to anesthetize him and then pour the rest on the spot where the bullet entered to disinfect it before they cut it out with a glowing hot knife blade? Those were the days when men were real men!

Alcohol works to destroy the proteins in the outer walls of germs, thus killing them on contact.

The takeaway from this section for you is to wash your hands several times a day and especially after you think you have been in a doctor's office or a clinic or even a big-box store or grocery store where many people have passed through. If it is cold or flu season, this tide of humanity will also be carrying a tidal wave of potentially infective microorganisms.

Your first line of defense should be to eradicate them from the surface of your hands as soon as possible before you invariably spread them to your face. This will do more than anything else I describe to lower your chances of becoming infected. Keep in mind, however, that hygiene, if taken too far, can be a double-edged sword that can actually impair your immunity. Let us take a look at how that works.

THE HYGIENE HYPOTHESIS

The hygiene hypothesis states that children are harmed immunologically when they are raised in an unnaturally, excessively clean environment. As bizarre and counterintuitive as that sounds, it is very true; here is why.

Children who grow up on farms, rolling around in animal manure and dirt all day, or those who grew up in filthy ghettos have much better immune systems than kids who don't. How could that be you ask?

Well-intentioned mothers are harming their children by constantly spraying disinfectants around them and cleaning every surface they touch. Those children wind up having skyrocketing rates of allergies, asthma, eczema, and infections from their poorly developed immunity. The reason being is that their immune systems are not being challenged by the usual sea of pathogens (germs) that accost us every day.

Repeated exposures to bacteria, viruses, and fungi are natural; and our body's immune system is perfectly designed to handle it. Those constant challenges are like lifting weights to your muscles—it builds a powerful robust immune system. Such a system has a vast storehouse of immunological memory that can be referenced whenever it encounters a pathogen. That is normal and a very good thing. The larger the library of germs recognized by your immune cells, the greater your immunity and the more robust your health.

Think about it: as a species, we began and evolved in a jungle environment, exposed to all sorts of pathogens, bitten by bugs of all types, drinking water that might not be very clean. Our bodies are designed to withstand all of that and to flourish. Don't mess with Mother Nature; we are perfectly designed.

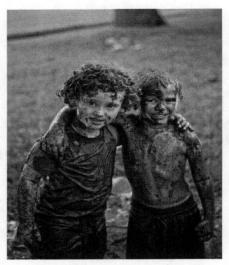

Let your kids be kids, rolling around in the dirt, eating it, playing with it, having the time of their lives. We are designed to eat butter and drink whole milk and eat animals from nose to tail, not sparing any parts. We are creatures that belong outside in the sunlight and fresh air and dirt for that matter. Do you think those boys in the above photo had a good time? Hell yeah, they did! What child remembers being clean and sanitized? None. And the beautiful part is those boys will be much healthier with less allergies, asthma, and skin problems. Sounds like a win-win to me.

NUTRITIONAL DEFICIENCIES AND YOUR IMMUNITY

Certain nutrients such as vitamins C and D and zinc are critical to maintaining a robust immunity. However, there are a host of other essential nutrients that should not be ignored.

Mineral deficiencies are often below the radar of the average patient. They are of supreme importance for your general health and critical to the function of your immune system. Enzymes and many vitamins will not work properly or at all if there are significant mineral deficiencies.

If you want your body to function properly and get all the nutrients it needs, you need to supplement magnesium, zinc, iodine, and selenium. Our soils are severely depleted of minerals and trace elements after seventy-five years of relentless chemical bombardment without the replacement of anything other than NPK (nitrogen, phosphorus, and potassium).

They have the utter audacity to describe NPK as a complete fertilizer, ignoring all the other minerals and trace elements that plants need to grow into healthy, nourishing foods. If you want to read more about this, I go into it in great detail in both my earlier books, *The Doomsday Book of Medicine* and *The Bible of Alternative Medicine*.

Magnesium alone is essential for the proper function of over three hundred enzymes, and zinc is responsible for another two hundred. That means by supplementing only zinc and magnesium, you will ensure the proper function of over five hundred enzymes essential for your health. If you still think that is not a big deal, then listen up.

Enzymes are essential. They speed up reactions in your body so it can properly function. They bind to their targets and turn them on so they can now do what your body needs. For example, digestive enzymes are released depending on the type of food that you have eaten. If your body is fed fat, it will release fat-digesting enzymes or lipases, amylases for starch digestion, and proteases for protein digestion. Enzymes only affect their target or substrate; they have no effect on anything else. They are specific for one molecule.

Enzymes are essential for the function of your digestion, respiration, muscle, and nerve function among many other of the body's roles.

Without enzymes, you will have no energy production, detoxification of dangerous substances, repairing of damaged body parts, and healing in general. Your blood pressure is controlled by enzymes. Your brain would not function at all without enzymes. If your brain dysfunction becomes severe enough, you could find yourself becoming "woke." Imagine that… The horror, the horror. However, yet once again, I digress.

Each enzyme is responsible for a specific function. What do you think happens when five hundred of your enzymes begin to malfunction? It is a huge catastrophe for your health. The reason people and most doctors do not recognize this is that it is a very slow process, and once the organs are damaged, the source of that damage is very elusive.

Trust me on this: supplement with zinc, magnesium, selenium, and iodine as a bare minimum. If you are more determined, then there are other supplements that provide all the minerals and trace elements your body needs. I like one called supreme fulvic. It has the complete complement of minerals and trace elements that your body needs for good health. It also contains both fulvic and humic acid complexes, which are great for your health, including opening up your cells so minerals and vitamins can more readily be absorbed.

You would normally get fulvic and humic complexes from eating a diet high in organic plants that are grown on ancient mineral rich soils. Certainly, that is not the state of the vast majority of our present farm soils. Hence, it is extremely difficult to get all the proper nutrition your body craves without supplementation.

Fulvic acid is found in large quantities in compost-rich soils. It is part of what is called the humic structure. It is made by the action of soil microbes on decaying plant matter in the presence of adequate oxygen. Fulvic acid carries over seventy different minerals and trace elements into our cells and is nature's way of processing decaying plant matter in a form that can be easily absorbed by the roots of living plants.

It is in a form that is easily recognized and absorbed by our bodies and carries a positive charge that makes it readily absorbed by the negatively charged intestinal lining.

Remember: opposite charges attract, and like charges repel. I know, you don't remember much from high school chemistry. Whoever thought it would come in handy? Now that is coming back to haunt you.

Now, what happens when you constantly poison soil with pesticides, herbicides, and fungicides and then use NPK chemical fertilizers? That soil is dead, devoid of microbial life that cannot break down plant matter and therefore cannot produce those vital fulvic and humic substances that are so essential for our health. That is why I strongly suggest you supplement both of them.

This I cannot emphasize emphatically enough: if the food you eat is grown on depleted, chemically poisoned, eroded soils, the plants grown from them will be devoid of many of the minerals, trace elements, and essential amino acids that your body needs to maintain good health!

Unfortunately, most doctors do not test for mineral deficiencies. Consequently, patients are blind as to their nutritional levels and needs. However, the vast majority of patients that I have treated in my thirty-seven years of practice have been both mineral and vitamin deficient—vitamin D and magnesium deficiencies being the most common.

Nobody summed up the situation better than two-time Nobel laureate Dr. Linus Pauling when he famously said, "One could trace every sickness, every disease and every ailment to a mineral deficiency."

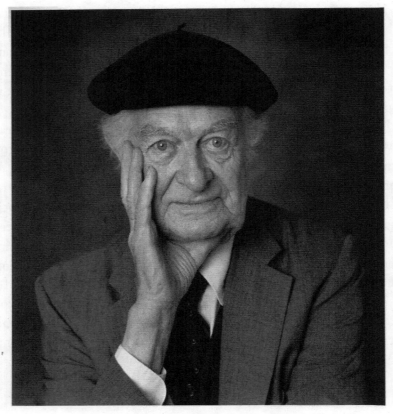

(Courtesy of Wikipedia)

A JUMP START FOR THE PREVENTION OF COLDS, FLU, COVID-19, AND ANY RESPIRATORY TRACT INFECTION

Later on in this book, I will take a much deeper dive into the actual treatments. This is just a quick reference that you can turn to if you feel one of these infections starting to "come on" and would like to stop it in its tracks.

VITAMIN C, VITAMIN D, AND ZINC

As a bare minimum, in order to jump-start my patients' immune systems and provide them with some protection, I use vitamins C, D, and zinc.

This is not the end point but rather the starting point of what I use. I build on this trio depending upon the patient's particular needs.

Strengthening your immunity will raise the wall that COVID-19 or any other microorganisms must overcome to infect you. In my humble opinion, it is your best bet at prevention.

This is my fourth decade practicing medicine, and I can assure you, without reservation, that boosting your immune system does work to both prevent and treat any infection, whatever the cause, including the much-feared (in my opinion, totally unwarranted) coronavirus. I have placed thousands of my patients on simple immune-boosting vitamin regimens, primarily vitamin C and vitamin D3 and zinc, with excellent results.

I always remind them that the vitamin D must be taken with fat to absorb it since it is fat soluble. The vitamin C is water soluble and thus can be taken on an empty stomach or with food. Zinc, like most minerals, is best absorbed with a meal.

Mimic nature as much as possible in your life. In nature, you would never have minerals and vitamins isolated in a single dose. They are always part of a complex plant or animal food. As such, they are mixed with fats; and their essential fatty acid components to help absorb fat-soluble vitamins, proteins, and their essential amino acids are complexed with various minerals and trace elements. Thus taking your iron with food that contains vitamin C will increase its absorption by 25 percent. Calcium and vitamin D work synergistically as well.

The list of these nutritional pairings is endless. The important takeaway is to take all your vitamins and minerals with food. In a pinch, you can take your B and C vitamins without anything since they are water soluble, and you always have water in your body. However, even they are better utilized and more bioavailable (meaning more readily absorbed and used by your body) when taken with a meal.

Many of my patients had been suffering with colds every "change of season," meaning the fall and spring. Once they were taking vitamin C, usually 1,000 mg or one gram daily, and 5,000 international units of vitamin D3 daily, and zinc 50 mg., most noted either having no infections; or if they did, they were very mild. This regimen is inexpensive, readily available, and has nothing but beneficial side effects. It is a very good starting point if you are not currently supplementing.

With the exception of hydroxychloroquine and ivermectin, the treatments in this book require no prescriptions. For that reason, it is essential that you stock up on all the treatments I mention. In a crisis, we have seen how store shelves become stripped of everything, including vitamins. Hydroxychloroquine and ivermectin were mentioned in the context of COVID-19 in an effort to highlight their efficacy.

Currently, with COVID-19, I have added chelated zinc about 50 mg daily with food. Chelated means it is bound to something, usually an amino acid that makes it much better absorbed. There will be two names on the zinc label indicating that it is chelated, names such as zinc picolinate, zinc methionine, zinc citrate, etc.

A mineral is inorganic and, as such, is not recognized by the body and thus is poorly absorbed. Once you chelate or combine an inorganic mineral such as zinc with an amino acid, it is now organic and much more easily absorbed and utilized by the body. Hence the reason for chelation of zinc and other minerals.

Cheap minerals are not chelated and are worthless. Don't bother taking them. I also have my patients take their mineral supplements with food as a way to further boost absorption. It is all about absorption. It doesn't matter how much of something you ingest; it is how much you absorb into your body that counts.

With the first sign of any infection, I would double the doses of all three of them. As your body is fighting off this infection, it utilizes massive amounts of antioxidants like vitamin C. Vitamin D is not an antioxidant, but it is essential for proper immune function.

For those reasons, I would keep increasing my vitamins C and D intake to stay ahead of the infection. You know you have saturated your body's vitamin C when you reach the limit of bowel tolerance and develop diarrhea. At that point, back off to your previous dose.

Vitamin D is now known to activate the immune system's T cells. T cells are like very effective assassins that eradicate viruses they come across in the blood, thus suppressing infections.

SUNSHINE AND YOUR HEALTH

We have known for centuries that sunshine helps cure tuberculosis and many viral diseases. For centuries, ill patients were encouraged to sit in the sun. Solariums were built on the roofs of hospitals and private clinics specifically to help cure TB patients. Low vitamin D levels are shown to be inversely proportional to your susceptibility to infection with colds, flu, and tuberculosis. That means it is like a see-saw effect—as vitamin D levels go down, respiratory infections are on the rise, and vice versa.

When you feel as if you are "coming down with something," boost your vitamin C, vitamin D, and zinc; and if possible, get yourself outside without sunblock in order to soak up some wonderful, healing sunlight.

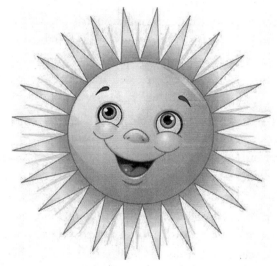

Once again, I have learned over the decades of studying medicine and the human body that if you mimic nature as close as you can, it has enormous health benefits. Go to sleep when the sun goes down, arise when it rises, walk barefoot on the grass, soak in the healing sun, eat lots of organic fruit and vegetables, eat free-range animals from nose to tail, include whole milk, eggs from free-range chickens, butter, and bone broth and you will experience endless benefits for your health and the well-being of your mind.

Medical history is full of examples of the use of sunlight to both prevent and cure diseases. Heat and sunlight are deadly to most germs that infect us, especially many viruses. The ultraviolet C component of sunshine is directly viricidal (deadly to viruses) and bacteria.

Have you ever noticed on small ponds they use a fountain to spray water high in the air? This is a very effective, inexpensive way to clean pond water by sterilization with the ultraviolet C component of sunlight? I even have an ultraviolet C generator in my private office where it sterilizes the room of pathogens every hour or so. Ultraviolet C machines are also used to sterilize airplanes/jets between flights.

About a third of the world's population has been infected with tuberculosis bacteria. However, the vast majority of which are in the third world and are exposed to sunlight all year round. Hence, they have very high levels of vitamin D circulating in their blood. Because of this, their immune systems are able to wall off the tuberculosis in what are known as granulomas. In other words, they do not have active tuberculosis, and thank God for that (among a host of many other reasons).

My point is that as a society, we are almost universally deficient in vitamin D from our "cave-dwelling" habits of remaining indoors almost exclusively. This is especially true of young people who are obsessed with computers, telephones, and television and rarely venture out of the doors. This not only eliminates all the wonderful benefits of vitamin D but also many other benefits of sunshine.

Unfortunately for them, as these young people age, they will have significantly more health problems than previous generations. They are obese from lack of exercise and are not developing strong bones, which comes from exercise, as well as calcium which is not absorbed without vitamin D. The diet of the average American is lacking in vitamins, minerals, and trace elements as well as essential fatty acids and essential amino acids. *Essential* means your body cannot produce them on its own, so it is essential that they be obtained in the food we eat.

Many of them live in environments that are constantly sanitized and sterilized, preventing their immune systems from being challenged and thus stunting its development, leaving them vulnerable to allergies, asthma, eczema, and many other medical problems.

You see, our immune systems "rise to the challenge" of attacks upon them by endless hordes of bacteria, viruses, and fungal invaders. That is what supercharges our immunity and allows it to develop an entire library of germs that it recognizes from having beaten them in the past.

Thus when exposed to any of them a second time, it immediately springs into action, cross-checking them against their stored memory. If it is a positive match, immediately, massive amounts of antibodies are produced, and this eradicates the invaders. This is why you are immune to infections you previously had such as measles, chicken pox, and thousands of others. It is a beautifully designed system.

Vaccines work to mimic natural infection by using proteins from a particular virus that trigger an immune response and then stores them in the immune system's memory bank. Subsequently, if the body recognizes the outer coat or capsid of the virus, it will immediately churn out millions of antibodies to defeat the invader and thus provide lasting immunity.

If we were not designed for that, we would have become extinct long ago. Don't listen to "the experts" who tell you otherwise. They are mistakenly warning patients who have had COVID-19 that their antibodies drop after about three months and thus are no longer immune and will need a vaccine. That is complete and utter nonsense, and they should know better.

The ultimate decline in antibody production is what always happens. Your body is beautifully designed. It reacts to an infection, produces antibodies for several months, and then once the infection subsides, it stores the memory in its B lymphocytes. If we kept making antibodies to every infection we were exposed to, our blood would be a thick sludge of antibodies to past infections that are no longer a threat.

That is ridiculous and would be totally inefficient, which our bodies clearly are nothing but. That is why vaccination of patients who have had COVID-19 is insane and, in my opinion, dangerous since you are introducing a foreign artificial mRNA along with a host of noxious chemicals and nanoparticles into a body that already has robust natural immunity that will immediately reference its immune memory and begin a counterattack!

I have encouraged the use of vitamin D among my patients who I universally check for its deficiency. I rarely find a patient who has adequate vitamin D levels. If I do, invariably, they are employed in a job that has them outside under the sun, such as construction workers, farmers, etc.

I have been personally using vitamin D for decades and prescribing it to my patients to prevent the types of respiratory tract infections that we are discussing in this chapter.

When COVID-19 broke out in early 2020, I immediately made vitamin D3 part of my specific recommendations for both its prevention and treatment. I watched closely as the "medical experts," both on television and in the medical literature, ignored vitamins C, D, and zinc. Then it finally happened; they noted that patients low on all three of them had much worse outcomes. Incredibly, they still did not recommend using them for either prevention or treatment.

Over the course of the last year or so, they have slowly come to the realization that all three are essential in its prevention and treatment. Once again woefully behind we underground medicine doctors, who appreciated the absolute necessity of supplementing with all three as a bare minimum. They mostly have focused on vitamin D and zinc, ignoring the most important vitamin C—but hell, at least it is some progress.

The bad news is that this information has not made its way to the docs "in the trenches," on the front lines treating their patients in hospitals, clinics, and private practices nationwide.

In conclusion, I would encourage all my readers to spend as much time in the sun and outdoors as they can. It can be done quite safely.

Old Yankee farmers from New England, although they were almost exclusively of English, Irish, Scottish, and German stock, had very deep healthy tans. This was because they were outside all year round. As the days got longer and the sun stronger, they already had a healthy base tan to protect their skin and did not have problems with sunburns, or skin cancer for that matter.

Sunburn and its inevitable cousin skin cancer is a modern-day phenomenon due to our living primarily indoors out of the healing sun. When we do venture out frequently, we overdo it and get sunburnt. Repeated sunburns lead to skin cancer, not sun exposure.

If you acclimate yourself getting a half an hour daily for the first week, then double it to an hour and so forth, you will not get burnt and you will have a nice healthy tan despite your skin tone. Naturally, if you are an albino, ignore that advice. Then again, other than Edgar Winter, when was the last time you saw an albino?

In my not-so-humble opinion, I think dermatologists have done an incredible disservice to America, with their constant admonishments about the dangers of sun exposure and the necessity of wearing sunblock to prevent melanoma. If sun exposure caused skin cancer, we would have gone extinct as a species long ago.

Also, one would expect that outdoor workers, such as construction workers, would have astronomical rates of melanoma, but the opposite is true. Their rates are low. Where are the rates the highest? Good question, grasshopper—among office workers! They are the ones who are inside cave dwellers all week, living under artificial lighting and venturing out only on weekend into the sun. Even stranger, most of their melanomas are in areas not exposed to the sun! Yet they keep pushing this insanity about the dangers of the sun.

There are other additional benefits of exposure to sunlight. Sunlight lowers your cholesterol levels since cholesterol is the backbone by which vitamin D is constructed. Blood pressure is also lowered by sunlight. And as if it couldn't get any better, sunlight also improves your mood. Hell, who doesn't feel better outside in nature on a beautiful sunny day?

Although there are exceptions to every rule, like my ex-wife for instance. No amount of sunshine improved her nasty disposition. All first marriages should be banned by law, just my humble opinion. However, once again, I digress. I have to confess my digressions are just so damn enjoyable!

In conclusion, if you feel you have been exposed to a respiratory tract infection, from close contact with someone infected, or if you feel the onset of cold symptoms, then you should immediately begin supplementation with vitamins C, D, and the mineral zinc. If this is a recurrent problem for you, then stay on all three for prevention.

If on all three you feel a respiratory tract infection "brewing," then immediately double your doses of vitamin C and D. Wait three days; if it's still a problem, then double them again. That will do more than anything else to help eradicate any impending infection. In the chapters ahead, I will teach you about the Gang of Seven and other ways that have emerged from the medical underground to treat any infection.

CHAPTER FIVE

BOOSTING YOUR IMMUNITY; THE 800 LB. GUERILLA THAT EVERYONE IS IGNORING

To my utter amazement, during this unprecedented coronavirus pandemic with COVID-19, there isn't any discussion of taking measures to boost the immune system. This chapter will teach you what to do for either a current infection or, more importantly, how to build an immune system that is as close to an impervious shield as *possible*. Nothing is absolute—you may still get an infection, but it will be shorter and much less serious if your immune system is *supercharged by using* my methods and other secrets from the medical underground.

There is universal acknowledgement that the coronavirus like all infections, only strikes those whose immune systems are overcome and defeated by the virus. Yet the health officials who are advising Americans only advise social distancing, handwashing, quarantine, and masks. Other than handwashing, all the other methods are minimally effective, if at all, in preventing the spread of most viruses, including COVID-19.

Those are the only defensive measures taken. Nobody is talking about boosting your immune system. It is a medical fact that certain nutrients such as vitamins and minerals and other nutraceuticals help boost our immune system. There are also many foods that work to boost our immunity. Yet the "experts" advising us are totally silent on this subject, even as their colleagues begin to die in substantial numbers from this infection.

As of the writing of this chapter, over forty physicians have died in Italy, and this is just beginning here in the United States. These doctors are not elderly. I have absolutely no information on their deaths, but my guess would be that they were not taking any measures to boost their immunity, were working long hours, were not eating well, were sleep deprived, and most likely had vitamin and zinc deficiencies or comorbidities (other illnesses)—a perfect storm for depressing one's immunity. Add to that significant and repeated viral exposure and you have forty dead docs.

When a virus "passes through" an area, not everyone exposed to it gets an infection. Why is that? The reason is the state of one's immune system. People with powerful immune systems are naturally resistant to infections. Even in the same family, often one member will fall ill while a spouse sharing the same bed will remain unaffected. Clearly, they had direct contact and significant exposure to their spouse's germs but remain untouched. That is no mystery; it is solely a consequence of the state of the other person's immune system.

Those with impaired immunity—whether as a consequence of starvation, general nutrient deficiencies, comorbidities (having other chronic diseases), or a decimated microbiome—are the people who get infected. That is the reason I want to teach you how to do what you can to move yourself into the category of those with natural "resistance" from a strong immune system. Let's see how best to do that.

IMMUNITY AND THE ANTIOXIDANT CASCADE

What are antioxidants? Antioxidants are substances that inhibit oxidation. Oxidation is a chemical reaction in the body that produces free radicals that damage the cells and organs of your body. Antioxidants neutralize those free radicals, thus preventing them from harming your body.

Antioxidants come in many forms, most of which are enzymes that your body produces, but many are vitamins and minerals such as vitamins A, C, and E (your ACE in the hole, so to speak), CoQ10, and lipoic acid and the mineral selenium. Zinc and iodine, while not technically antioxidant minerals, do have amazing benefits for your immunity. Many foods are very high in antioxidants and are wonderful for our health and as such are called superfoods.

One of the easiest ways to boost your immunity is via the antioxidant cascade. This concept was popularized by Dr. Lester Packer at the University of California. In a nutshell, Dr. Packer discovered in his research that certain vitamins are so important to immunity that they regenerate each other. On the fat-soluble side, vitamin E and CoQ10 regenerate each other, and on the water-soluble side, vitamin C and glutathione regenerate one another.

Incredibly, there is only one substance that is both fat and water soluble, and that is alpha lipoic acid (also sometimes called lipoic acid). As you might have guessed, it regenerates both the fat- and water-soluble antioxidants, therefore recharging both the fat- and water-soluble branches of your immune system.

Previously, you couldn't take glutathione orally since it was destroyed in the stomach. There are now forms of glutathione that can be either taken orally or via suppository (placed in your rectum). The oral form is known as liposomal glutathione, and as the name implies, it is wrapped in a lipid or fat layer called a phospholipid complex, which prevents its degradation in your stomach and allows it to be absorbed in your small intestine. Call me crazy, but I will go with the oral preparation.

Therefore if you take liposomal glutathione, vitamin C, CoQ10, vitamin E, and alpha lipoic acid (or lipoic acid) you are going a long way to boosting your overall immunity. Now, this is a simplified version of Dr. Packer's research, which is much more involved than stated here. But for our purposes, this will suffice.

FOODS THAT SUPPORT YOUR IMMUNITY

It is always preferable to get your medicine from your food. Nutritious food is always superior to synthetic medicines simply because of all the beneficial nutrients present in foods. Processed foods are devoid of most of the beneficial substances naturally present in food due to the manufacturing process and other factors.

Many of the foods that provide high doses of antioxidants are preferably eaten raw, since the heat of cooking destroys both antioxidant vitamins, minerals, and enzymes. That is not an ironclad rule. Sometimes, cooking methods like fermentation help increase the nutrition in a food.

High-antioxidant-containing foods such as fresh fruits and vegetables (preferably organic) are a great way to boost your immune system. Your body recognizes these foods and readily absorbs and assimilates them without having to go through the steps of detoxification in the liver.

Nonorganic foods are laced with herbicides, pesticides, fungicides, and chemical fertilizers that your body has to detoxify via complex chemical processes, primarily in your liver. This is a burden for your liver that is not there with organic foods. Who in their right mind wants to ingest all those harmful, cancer-causing chemicals if given the choice?

One of the primary harmful effects of a processed, chemical-laden diet is its effect on your gut bacteria. The bacteria in your gut are part of the very large family of thousands of species of bacteria, fungi, and even viruses that, in their totality, make up what is known as your microbiome.

Your microbiome overall, and especially in your gut or gastrointestinal tract are the front-line troops of your immune army. I will go into a deeper explanation of their role in immunity at the end of this chapter.

We all remember the warm, healthy feeling one has after eating a hearty bone broth or chicken soup. Chicken soup is a staple among Americans for many generations, and for a good reason. It is a powerhouse of nutrition and helps enhance your immunity. It provides amino acids, vitamins, minerals that all help your immunity and promote healing. As a medicine, it tastes great and comes highly recommended by my mother!

Bone broth is another wonderfully nutritious food that, without a doubt, you should make part of your diet. Not only is it a powerful source of collagen, but it also contains healthy fats, vitamins, minerals, and trace elements.

Antioxidants-for-Health-and-Longevity

Antioxidant	Primary Benefits Or Function (in addition to general antioxidant benefits)	Sources (bold items are best)
NETWORK ANTIOXIDANTS — The most significant antioxidants; these work together synergistically		
Vitamin C	cardiovascular, joints, cancer prevention, vision, liver, acne, Alzheimer's, asthma, depression, diabetes, Parkinson's and more...	**raw peppers, parsley, broccoli, cauliflower, citrus fruits, berries, romaine lettuce, brussels sprouts, papaya, cantaloupe,** and many more...
Vitamin E	heart and circulatory system, many other benefits as well	**mixed-tocopherol vitamin E supplements** sunflower seeds, almonds, greens
Coenzyme Q-10	heart and circulatory system, gums, blood sugar regulation, cellular energy	**CoQ-10/ubiquinol supplements** fish, organ meats
Glutathione	energy, respiratory system, vision, immunity	**spinach, potatoes, asparagus, avocado, squash, okra, cauliflower, broccoli, walnuts, garlic**
Alpha-Lipoic Acid	vision, diabetes	**alpha-lipoic acid supplements,** broccoli, spinach, and other green leafy vegetables, organ meats
Selenium	Supports and replenishes all of the network antioxidants	**Brazil nuts, selenium supplements,** cod, shrimp, snapper, tuna, halibut, calves' liver, sardines, salmon
CAROTENOIDS — a family of plant pigments that work in combination to provide powerful antiaging benefits. Eat with fats.		
Vitamin A Beta Carotene	heart disease, cancer, respiratory and immune system, skin and joints, vision, arthritis, diabetes, protection from radiation	**chlorella, spirulina and other green superfoods, dark green leafy vegetables, cooked carrots, pumpkin, sweet potatoes,** cantaloupe, squash
Lutein and Zeaxanthin	vision — prevention of cataracts and macular degeneration	**cooked greens, green peas,** romaine, brussels sprouts, corn, broccoli
Lycopene	heart disease, cancer prevention (esp. prostate), vision, exercise-induced asthma	**cooked tomatoes** watermelon, guava, raw tomatoes, pink grapefruit
Astaxanthin	joint pain, inflammation, vision, brain and nervous system, stamina, skin, many more...	**astaxanthin supplements** salmon, shrimp
BIOFLAVONOIDS — phytonutrients (plant chemicals); all useful as antioxidants, antivirals, and anti-inflammatories.		
Flavonoids	cardiovascular, asthma and allergies, vision, skin, gum disease	**virtually all fruits, vegetables, dry beans, green tea and other herbs and spices**
Quercetin	anti-inflammatory, anti-histamine, allergies, circulatory system, cancer prevention	**onions, chives, leeks, scallions, garlic,** most other fruits and vegetables
Rutin & Hesperidin	circulation, varicose veins, skin, allergies, vision, anti-inflammatory	**apricots, buckwheat, cherries, prunes, rose hips, the rind of citrus fruits**
Curcumin	inflammation, cancer prevention, anti-bacterial, cardiovascular, nervous system	**turmeric, curcumin supplements**
Ginkgo Biloba	circulation, brain function, memory, vision	**ginkgo biloba supplements**
Anthocyanins	circulation, vision, brain function	**acai, goji berries, mangosteen, noni,** berries
Pycnogenol	joint pain, circulation, skin, immune system	**pycnogenol supplements**
Resveratrol	cardiovascular system, life-extension, cancer prevention, immune system	**muscadine grape seeds and skin, resveratrol supplements,** organic red wine
Bilberry	vision, esp. night blindness, circulation	**bilberries, bilberry supplements**
Milk Thistle	liver detoxifier, boosts glutathione	**milk thistle supplements**

That wonderful chart is complements of fitbodybuzz.com.

In almost all cultures, except for ours, out of necessity, people did not waste anything. The carcass or bones were immediately made into a nutritious bone broth. They literally ate from nose to tail, including organ meats. The liver of any animal is a nutritional powerhouse, and they were always eaten, as were other organs such as spleen, heart, brain, and kidneys. Collectively, these organs are known as offal. Every society on earth, except ours, ate offal for its amazing nutritional benefits.

Liver, for example, provides much more nutrition than muscle meats. Liver is jam-packed with essential amino acids and whole proteins such as collagen, minerals, and vitamins, especially vitamins A and B12 and other B vitamins. It is a nutrient-dense superfood, and I recommend eating it on a regular basis, especially if you are pregnant.

We would be wise to adopt such eating habits. They are used by every culture for a reason. In addition, ecologically, it is incredibly efficient and non-wasteful. You can make all the arguments you want against eating animal products, but we are omnivores (meaning we eat plants as well as animal products) and, as such, are designed to sit atop the food chain and enjoy the amazing assortment of food available to us.

I love meat and fish, and as an omnivore, I will happily eat anything I want on the food chain. That is my gripe against people who try to impose their will on others because they don't agree with them. This is just censorship of others' opinions, primarily because they cannot hope to defeat them in a debate of ideas. If you want to be a vegetarian or a vegan or whatever, that is your choice. I couldn't care less, but don't give me a hard time because I love meat and fish. You have absolutely no right to impose your dietary choices on anyone else, despite what your liberal friends *have told you*!

On our college and university campuses, this madness is in full bloom, with the left censoring all conflicting opinions as hate speech. This is very convenient for them but disastrous for the students who are being indoctrinated, not educated. Our society as a whole and especially our schools should be *forums* of open, active debating of conflicting opinions, a marketplace of ideas, not reeducation camps for the left.

Fermented foods are another example of foods that are nutritionally dense, meaning chock-full of nutrients as well as probiotic bacteria. They are wonderful for your gut bacteria (your microbiome), aiding in digestion, boosting your immunity, and cutting sugar cravings. In fact, the traditional diets that I have described all enhance and nourish the microbiome in your gut. Many of the foods contain prebiotics that help feed the probiotic bacteria of your microbiome.

Every culture worldwide utilizes fermentation of different foods, for both a means of preservation and as a source of nutritional superfoods. Once again, the standard American diet is almost completely devoid of fermented foods. If you ever wanted to create a diet that would ruin someone's health, it is our current diet. It is loaded with sugar; empty calories devoid of nutrition; lacking in enzymes, vitamins, minerals, phytonutrients (plant nutrients) and trace elements. While at the same time it is chock-full of health-destroying chemicals, such as pesticides, herbicides, fungicides, heavy metals, and pollutants of all kinds. The consequences of this diet are seen in our skyrocketing cases of obesity, infertility, chronic diseases, and sadly, mental illness. Many of the most recent studies incredibly confirm the role of the damaged microbiome as the root cause of all of these conditions.

Centuries before the invention of refrigeration, out of necessity, all cultures turned to fermentation. They fermented a wide variety of different foods including fish, soybeans, bean curd, coconut water, and even pineapple juice.

A few examples of fermented foods are sauerkraut, yogurt, some cheeses, kimchi, kefir, kombucha, and pickles. Only some pickles are fermented, they say naturally fermented on their labels. The others are fermented using vinegar or sometimes lemon juice. Those pickles do not have the health benefits conferred by *true* fermentation.

The Italians and the Vietnamese traditionally ferment my personal favorite: anchovies. Nobody is on the fence about anchovies, either you love them or hate them. I eat them right out of the bottle, grossing out my wife.

VITAMIN C

Let's take a deep dive into the king of antioxidants and immune support: vitamin C or ascorbic acid. If you had to make a choice of one vitamin to take, then hands down vitamin C is the winner. Thank God that is not a choice we have to make, but given the scary nature of recent times, you never know. The good news is that it is inexpensive, almost totally devoid of side effects, and readily available for most Americans.

Vitamin C was first brought to the attention of the American public by the only two-time Nobel-prize winner Linus Pauling when he wrote *Vitamin C and the Common Cold*. I read this book in college, and it literally changed my life, starting me on a path of exploration of nutrition for not just the prevention but also for the treatment of disease.

Dr. Pauling's famous quote still rings true today: "You can trace every sickness, every disease, and every ailment to a mineral deficiency."

Dr. Pauling was a brilliant biochemist, and as such, he understood that vitamins do not work without minerals, which act as cofactors, enabling their function. Hence if you are deficient in minerals and trace elements, then even if you have adequate vitamin intake, they will not function properly.

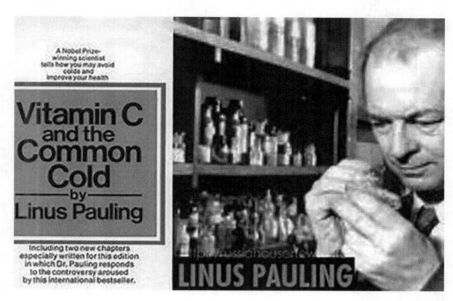

As I touched on earlier, vitamin C is a water-soluble vitamin (along with all the B vitamins). Since it is water soluble, it does not have to be taken with food or fat and thus can be taken on an empty stomach, since our bodies are approximately 60 percent water.

Vitamin C comes in various forms: Ascorbic acid, which has a sour taste to it. Another form is sodium ascorbate, which does not have that sour taste. Emergen-C is a brand name of a powdered form of vitamin C; it has mixed ascorbates (various types of vitamin C) as well as B vitamins and minerals such as manganese, zinc, and chromium as well as electrolytes. All of which support your immune system.

There is a man-made version of vitamin C that is fat soluble, known as liposomal vitamin C. Liposomal means it is wrapped in a phospholipid (fat) envelope, thus making it fat soluble. It is much better absorbed than water-soluble versions of vitamin C. It binds to the enterocytes (the cells lining the intestine) and, from there, goes to the liver and into the bloodstream; and from the blood, it is able to cross the cell wall and enter your cells. The difference in absorption is considerable: 93 percent for liposomal vs. 19 percent for water-soluble vitamin C.

The amazingly high absorption levels of liposomal vitamin C make it comparable to intravenous administration, which has 100 percent absorption. Unlike normal *water-soluble* vitamin C, which is not stored in the body and any not *utilized is* eliminated in your urine. Liposomal vitamin C, on the other hand, is fat soluble, hence it is stored in your fat and not eliminated in your urine.

Vitamin C is amazingly nontoxic—in fact, it is less toxic than water! The only side effect from too much vitamin C orally is diarrhea. That is known as bowel tolerance. If you are titrating up (taking progressively higher doses) your vitamin C because of an illness or other reason and you develop diarrhea, then just lower your dose to your previous dose that your bowels can tolerate, and the diarrhea should abate. Hence the term *bowel tolerance.*

Vitamin C works against infections by supporting your immune system. It does so by supercharging your body's white cells by being directly antiviral. It does this by directly inactivating the RNA or DNA of the specific virus, thus preventing the virus from replicating (reproducing).

Vitamin C also increases the production of interferon, which prevents cells from being invaded by a virus. When cells are infected with a virus, they release interferon (which is a signaling protein) that does two things: it interferes with viral replication (thus its name), and it prevents the virus from invading nearby cells. Hence you can see how critical adequate vitamin C levels are for treatment and prevention of all viral infections.

Vitamin C supercharges many of the components of the immune system. It regenerates glutathione while also acting as a strong antioxidant and finally by squelching the cytokine storm produced by infections that is so damaging and often fatal. The cytokine storm is responsible for the death of many patients infected with COVID-19.

HOW TO DOSE YOUR VITAMIN C

Vitamin C dosing depends on if you are sick or healthy. If you are healthy, I recommend 1,000 mg or 1 gram twice a day. If you are taking liposomal vitamin C, then 1,200 mg once a day with a fatty meal should suffice.

If you are sick, I recommend steadily increasing your vitamin C by doubling it every two or three days, to bowel tolerance. If that occurs, lower it to the previous dose. As any illness progresses, the body's vitamin C requirements skyrocket.

If you are sick with the COVID-19 virus, I highly recommend taking liposomal vitamin C since its absorption is comparable to intravenous vitamin C, and thus your blood levels will be high. I would take between 8 and 12 grams of liposomal a day. You should note, there is no problem taking both forms of vitamin C.

For regular (non-liposomal) ascorbic acid you may find yourself doubling it until you are taking 20 to 30 grams a day orally. But you will probably reach bowel tolerance well before that time. Certainly, intravenous is the best way to get it, but that often is not available.

Remember the immune cascade that I was teaching you about earlier? Vitamin C regenerates glutathione, which is the strongest antioxidant and detoxifier in the body, thus also helping boost your immunity.

Vitamin C has also been shown time and time again to be universally lethal to all viruses. This lethality depends on the dose and the method of administration, with intravenous naturally being the king. A wonderful source of all thing vitamin C is the website Orthomolecular.org. It has the most complete and up-to-date information on using vitamin C to treat disease and other fascinating topics in orthomolecular medicine, which I fully endorse.

The mainstream media and traditional medicine often mistakenly describe the use of vitamins, minerals, and nutraceuticals as being unsupported by research and therefore without any validity. This website easily refutes that fake news. It is chock-full of peer-reviewed studies, meta-analyses, and articles supporting its concepts.

High vitamin C–containing foods include the well-known citrus fruits such as oranges, lemons, limes, also turnip greens, swiss chard, kale, sweet peppers, guava, kiwi, broccoli, strawberries, pineapple, papaya, mango, cauliflower, grapefruit, cantaloupe, black currants, and sun-dried tomatoes. Potatoes are also a good source of vitamin C and also potassium. Don't overcook them and leave the skins on to retain more of the vitamin C.

VITAMIN D3

Vitamin D3 is more like a hormone than a vitamin. That means it acts as a messenger to other parts of the body. It has numerous health-enhancing effects, and as research continues, we continuously learn of more and more benefits.

As humans, we are designed to have high vitamin D levels from our exposure to sunlight. Up until the last fifty years or so, most Americans played outdoors as children and worked outdoors. Thus their vitamin D levels were much greater than modern Americans, most of whom work inside and, now due to our obsession with computers, also play inside.

When children do go outside these days, their mothers are so paranoid about them getting skin cancer that they slather them with sunblock, thus preventing their limited exposure from generating vitamin D.

People of color have a built-in sunblock; the darker they are, the stronger that is. It is called melanin. Melanin is the pigment that gives your skin, hair, and the iris of your eyes its color. The darker you are, the more melanin you have.

Allow me to digress for a moment. Sunlight is wonderful for your health. It produces much-needed vitamin D, lowers your blood pressure, improves mood, increases calcium absorption, and lowers cholesterol. Cholesterol is the molecule that is the backbone for the vitamin D molecule, thus the production of vitamin D lowers your cholesterol.

Sunburns are bad for you and lead to skin cancer, not sunlight. My dermatologist colleagues have this one all wrong. Think about it, would nature design us to die of skin cancer if we were exposed to sunlight? Of course not. We would have gone extinct a long time ago.

What nature does do is produce more melanin for those who live in areas of more sunlight and less in others. This prevents the recurrent sunburns, which lead to cancer. After all, we are the naked apes as compared to our close relatives.

If evolution made us vulnerable to chronic sun exposure, we would have lost the trait of not having fur, and we would have devolved back to being hairy.

However, the opposite is true; since more of our skin was not covered with hair, it was directly exposed to sunlight and thus able to produce a lot of vitamin D, which by design is critically important to our immune system, absorbing calcium to build strong bones and grow tall, improve our mood, prevents colds, flu, and respiratory viruses such as coronavirus.

Studies are now showing that adequate levels of vitamin D may reduce your incidence of stroke, heart disease, and cancer among its other myriad benefits.

It is believed vitamin D improves mood by its effect on serotonin levels, which it increases. It also may play a direct role in helping SAD (seasonal affective disorder) and depression. Why do you think going outside on a beautiful day always makes you feel so good? Coincidence? I think not.

Guess what happens when you give patients with SAD some vitamin D? You are a genius! Now you have heard that from someone else besides your mother! Yes, grasshopper, it improves their mood and condition.

Vitamin D can directly kill viruses it meets. Studies have confirmed that it activates the body's T cells, decreases the production of pro-inflammatory cytokines, and boosts immunity.

Keep in mind that vitamin D is fat soluble, so as such, you need to take it with fat or you won't absorb it, and it is also stored in your fat. Studies done on American submariners (sailors on submarines) show that after three months of submersion without sunlight, they had completely depleted any vitamin D stored in their fat and had to begin supplementation to maintain their health.

Proof of the supreme importance of vitamin D in boosting your immunity and preventing viral infections comes every year with the advent of flu season.

Most Americans don't get much sunlight/vitamin D after September of each year. We know from the sailor studies that after three months, most Americans will have abysmally low vitamin D levels (that is assuming they had normal levels to start with, which is not the norm).

There is most certainly a flu season in the United States, which typically runs from December through March. It is no coincidence that December is three months after September, just about the time most people's vitamin D levels bottom out. By February, the pool of available people peaks and then dwindles into March and disappears altogether as the population ventures outside again in spring.

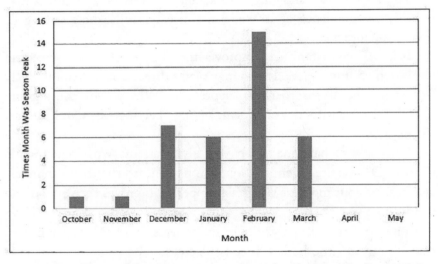

The CDC's own flu chart mirrors that of progressively diminishing vitamin D levels in our population. Still don't believe me?

Flu season among our cousins Down Under, in Australia, is the complete opposite of ours since their seasons are also the opposite. In other words, their time of warmth and sun exposure is during our winter. Their flu season is just the opposite of our own. And at the equator, it is all year round!

Why vitamin D3 is the best form of vitamin D for you to take: Vitamin D3 or cholecalciferol is the same form your body produces when it is exposed to sunlight. It is therefore what your body is designed to recognize and utilize, and it also lasts longer in your fat stores.

Vitamin D3 also comes from animal sources such as oily fish, liver, cheese, and eggs. Beef liver is a good source as is cod liver oil. Vitamin D2 comes from plant sources. One good way to get this form if you are desperate to get vitamin D is to place mushrooms upside down in the sun, gills up for several hours and they will produce vitamin D.

Sun exposure is preferable to any other way of getting your vitamin D. The ultraviolet B waves in natural sunshine striking your skin produces vitamin D3.

You should stay in the sun daily until it turns its first shade of pink, then get out of it. Naturally, this is for Whites and is without the use of sunblock. If you do this daily, starting in early spring, no matter how fair you are, you will develop a nice tan over the course of the season. You will never look as good as an Italian, but hey, you can dream, can't you?

Encourage your children to get out of the house and into the sun using the same system. This will ensure that they grow strong healthy bones and a good immune system and are in better moods!

There are conflicting reports as to the best latitudes to live at in the United States to get adequate vitamin D production from sunlight. From Thanksgiving to Easter, most of the United States above the Carolinas will not have strong-enough sunlight to produce vitamin D.

Below that level, you are good all year round. During the summer months with nothing but a bathing suit on (I personally prefer nude sunbathing, but I live isolated on a farm) and no sunblock, you will get 10,000 to 20,000 units of vitamin D3 every hour. The range is due to skin color—the darker your skin, the longer it will take.

Before I get to its dosing, one final note on vitamin D. The levels that most doctors go by are inadequate, the usual cutoff is a level of 30 ng/ml whereas the ideal level you need is between 60 ng/ml and 80 ng/ml. I like it closer to 80.

HOW TO DOSE YOUR VITAMIN D3

Normally, I advise my patients to take between 5,000 and 7,500 international units of vitamin D3 daily, with a fatty meal to ensure its absorption. If they go outside a lot during the nice-weather months or if they work outside, I will tell them to start it when the leaves drop and stop it when they come back out.

If you are sick with the flu or coronavirus, then I significantly raise the dose. If you test positive for either one, take 50,000 units of vitamin D3 daily for four days and then twice a week thereafter until you feel fully recovered. Remember to take it with fat. Don't wait until you are really sick. As soon as you start to feel punky, start your vitamin D3. There is no downside to that and plenty of upside.

If you have the flu or coronavirus and the weather is okay, get outside into the sun—you will feel better, and the ultraviolet light will help disinfect any virus that is exposed to it.

Finally, for COVID-19 science is slowly coming around and recommending vitamin D for both prevention and treatment. But trust me, this is currently a fringe opinion in early 2021. They also have seen the importance of zinc, without which hydroxychloroquine is totally ineffective. More on that later on. Only a few researchers have made the vitamin C connection.

I think one of the primary reasons for that is that they don't recognize its universal lethality to all viruses, including coronavirus or COVID-19 in this case. The ever-clever Chinese have recognized it and utilized it to great success in several hospitals. There are a few-forward thinking hospitals in the United States also using it.

Remember, vitamin D is fat soluble, so you will need to take it with a fatty meal. Anything fried counts—pizza, meats, dairy, and all oils. Oils are liquid fats at room temperature. Not taking it with fat is a waste of time since you will not absorb it. It doesn't matter what you take for quantity of any vitamin or supplement, it is what your body absorbs. The rest goes out as waste.

Another way to increase the absorption of vitamin D is with the use of magnesium. Magnesium helps increase the absorption of vitamin D and helps regulate its blood levels. Magnesium is a wonder element, with over three hundred enzymes requiring it to function properly. It helps lower blood pressure; treats abnormal heart rhythms, palpitations, muscle cramps, and spasms; and even relieves constipation.

Great natural sources of magnesium are dark green leafy vegetables and all types of nuts. Anything green has magnesium in it. The reason for that is the color green in plants is derived from chlorophyll, the central mineral of which is magnesium.

Fascinating is the fact that hemoglobin, the oxygen-carrying protein in human blood, is exactly the same as chlorophyll, but with iron as the central mineral. I always thought that was really cool, but then again, I thought the TV show *Alf* was hilarious. So much for my taste.

COQ10

Hopefully, you recall from my earlier discussion of immunity and the antioxidant cascade the importance of CoQ10. Coenzyme Q10 is part of the fat-soluble arm along with vitamin E that regenerate each other and, in turn, are both regenerated by alpha-lipoic acid. The human body is able to make its own CoQ10, that is why it is not considered an essential vitamin. However, it markedly diminishes as we age, thus the lack of energy in the elderly (among other reasons, primary being chronic dehydration). CoQ10 production also diminishes with chronic diseases such as diabetes and heart disease.

CoQ10 is a fat-soluble compound made by your body and stored in its mitochondria. The mitochondria are the powerhouses of the cell, responsible for its energy production. Thus the importance of CoQ10 to help produce energy and to support your immune system.

By far, the most common cause of low CoQ10 in patients is from the use of statin drugs that lower cholesterol. These drugs directly inhibit the body's pathway to produce CoQ10, yet amazingly, most cardiologists and primary care doctors still don't recommend its supplementation.

CoQ10 is concentrated in the organs of the body since they require large amounts of energy to properly function, hence eating organ meats such as liver, heart, etc., are excellent sources. Other sources are seafood and chicken. Vegetable sources include avocado, broccoli, cauliflower, nuts, and seeds.

DOSAGE OF COQ10

The usual dose of CoQ10 that I advise my patients to take—either for energy, immune support, or if they are currently on statin drugs—is 200 mg once a day. Remember, it is a fat-soluble substance, and as such, it needs to be taken with fatty food so it will be properly absorbed.

If you are eating and you are not sure of the fat content of your meal, you could add an oil to your salad to provide the fat you need. All oils are just liquid fats at room temperature—EVOO or extra virgin olive oil being the king of oils.

If you take one thing from this book, understand this fact: Fat is not your enemy; fat does not make you fat. Carbohydrates make you fat. Fats are essential for your health and, as such, are cleverly named essential fatty acids. Proteins are also essential, thus the essential amino acids. Notice there are no essential carbohydrates. You don't even need them in your diet to be healthy. Your body can fabricate the carbs it needs by a process known as gluconeogenesis. Boy, is that a mouthful.

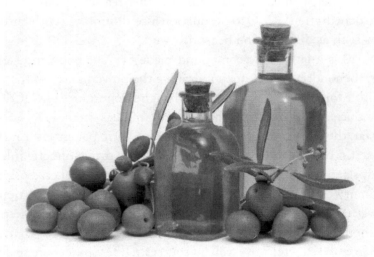

The healthiest diet is full of healthy fats of all kinds—butter, cheese, avocado, coconut, whole milk, lard, and other animal fats. Without healthy fat, you would become very ill in a short time. There are bad fats such as trans fats, no disrespect to the LGBTQ folks! Trans fats do the opposite of saturated fatty acids—they lower good HDL cholesterol and raise bad LDL cholesterol. They increase inflammation in the body, which never is a good thing. This in turn increases the risk of heart disease, diabetes, and stroke to name but a few.

Here are some of the health benefits of using a healthy oil such as olive oil. Seventy three percent of the of the fats in olive oil are monounsaturated fatty acids. This means they are stable in high heat, so you can use olive oil in cooking without destroying its healthy benefits. Oleic acid also lowers inflammation, and it is thought that it might also help regulate genes that cause cancer.

Olive oil has vitamins E and K, but more importantly, it is loaded with antioxidants. Olive oil might also be beneficial in preventing Alzheimer's disease, but I forget why. Only kidding! It is believed it does so by reducing the beta amyloid plaques that are produced in Alzheimer's. Olive oil also has antibacterial properties and appears to work against the bacteria *Helicobacter pylori*, which causes ulcers.

One study showed that 30 grams of EVOO daily for two weeks cured up to 40 percent of the patients. It also seems to work against antibiotic-resistant strains of this bacteria.

However, if you want to boost your immune system, I would double or even triple your daily intake. That will ensure that you are supercharging the fat-soluble wing of your antioxidants.

VITAMIN E

As I taught you earlier, the fat-soluble arm of the antioxidant cascade involves CoQ10 and vitamin E, which regenerate one another and, in turn, are both regenerated by alpha-lipoic acid. Vitamin E is also essential for proper human growth, fertility, immune function, central nervous system development, and muscle development. It is also essential to your vision and the health of your brain, skin, and even your blood.

Without vitamin E, all the fat in our body, including the membranes around all our cells, would turn rancid. Vitamin E does this by neutralizing toxic oxidants (acting as an antioxidant), thus preventing oxidation of the fat in our cell membranes.

Vitamin E is a fat-soluble vitamin and, as such, obviously needs to be taken with a meal containing fat so it can be properly absorbed.

The reason I keep mentioning solubility is because if you ignore it, the substance will pass right through you unabsorbed, and you will miss all its benefits.

What is the point of taking something that you are not going to gain any benefit from? I have been in practice over thirty-five years, and many times, a new patient will brag to me about their knowledge of vitamins, and they have taken them for decades. Almost every time they had been taking them on an empty stomach, not absorbing anything from them, except for vitamins B and C. They are water soluble and thus absorbed with or without food.

The flip side of water solubility is that there is nowhere to store them and have to be constantly replenished. Whereas the fat-soluble vitamins will store in your fat and can be drawn upon for months. Hence the wonderful benefits of sun exposure, which will produce prodigious amounts of vitamin D that you can store for future needs. The same holds true with all fat-soluble substances.

The downside of fat solubility is toxicity. If you can store it, you can store too much of it and they can become toxic, but that is rarely the case. Fat deficiencies are more common due to our fascination with low-fat diets.

If obesity is your problem or concern, then by all means dump as many of the carbs as you reasonably can. Personally, I think I could give them all up, except I have to have crusty bread with seeds in the crust with globs of real butter. My alternative food fantasy is same bread with a tasty virgin olive oil… Oh my god.

I have a patient from Portugal, Enrique Garcia, who has an olive orchard there and travels back and forth. He has the best olive oil I have ever tasted. It is fruity and absolutely delicious, and I am a connoisseur of olive oil. He brings me a bottle every year, and I treasure it.

Since vitamin E is fat-soluble, it will naturally be stored in your body's fat. However, it is found in the greatest quantities in male testes and in the uterus of females. Remember, nature never does anything by mistake. Vitamin E is critical to fertility, hence it is found in large quantities in our organs involved with reproduction. Vitamin E along with adequate iodine and enough saturated animal fats goes a long way toward correcting fertility problems.

Let's take a deep dive into the different types of vitamin E currently on the market. Vitamin E currently comes in eight different plant-derived forms and can get quite confusing for the layperson. There are two main subfamilies of vitamin E, tocopherols and tocotrienols, each with four members: designated alpha, beta, gamma, and delta.

The tocopherols are all closely related and, for our purposes, are all biologically active, meaning they work in our bodies. The designations of alpha, beta, etc., are in order of their potency or strength, with alpha being the strongest.

The tocotrienols are also quite useful and help our body in many ways. They help prevent cancers of various types including breast and prostate, as well as helping protect our nervous system.

Both subfamilies of vitamin E are beneficial for your health, and mixtures of each type are the best to take since they act synergistically (work together better than apart). However, when supplementing, they are best taken separately since tocopherols will interfere with the uptake of tocotrienols. The best form to take your vitamin E is natural mixed tocopherols, and natural mixed tocotrienols (separately).

There are also synthetic forms of vitamin E available, such as DL-alpha-tocopherol. The *l* after the *d* is the designation for synthetic. Avoid this form if you can since it is the least effective form. However, if you have nothing else, it will have to suffice.

The synthetic forms do not appear to cross the blood-brain barrier and, thus, do not enter your brain. They also do not appear to be able to enter your mitochondria of your cells where all the activity of the vitamin E takes place. So, stick with the natural forms for better absorption and biological activity.

There is another form of vitamin E currently on the market, which is an esterified vitamin E or ester-E. This form is lacking much of the biological activity of natural vitamin E and thus is not effective as an antioxidant and does not do well in preventing clots for example.

Since our goal is to boost our immune system, we will be taking a much higher dose of vitamin E and for a short time (until the infection has passed). The doses I am recommending should not be taken daily for long periods—you will develop toxicity.

You can also get a lot of natural, wholesome, easily absorbed vitamin E from your diet.

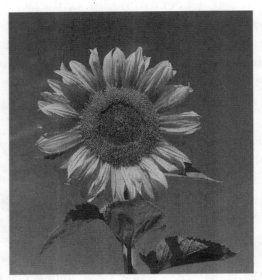

Foods such as green leafy vegetables, sunflower seeds, and nuts are excellent sources of vitamin E. You can also get both forms of vitamin E from coconut, palm, and rice bran oils. But like I said earlier, when you combine the two forms, the alpha-tocopherols may inhibit the uptake of tocotrienols.

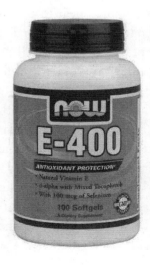

DOSING OF VITAMIN E

What I would suggest during an active infection is to take vitamin E with mixed natural tocopherols, 400 international units (that is how vitamin E comes), twice a day with a fatty meal. That should supply your body with all the vitamin E it needs to boost your immunity and suppress the infection.

If you have a serious infection, double it to 800 international units twice a day with fat. Once the infection passes, you must lower it to 400 international units once daily; otherwise, you run the risk of developing toxicity.

Toxicity can develop with any fat-soluble vitamin, such as vitamins A, D, E, and K since they are stored in your fat and not excreted in your urine like water-soluble vitamins.

IODINE

Iodine is an element that is essential for human health and survival. Without iodine, the human body cannot exist. Every cell in the body requires iodine and benefits from it. Iodine is especially concentrated in certain organs, such as the breast, thyroid, prostate, and ovaries.

Although it is not widely recognized by modern medicine, patients with cancers in those organs almost universally are severely deficient in iodine. Cysts in any of those same organs also are from an iodine deficiency, although you will never see that in medical textbooks. They attribute most cysts to either an infection or an obstructing duct. That is wrong. Iodine deficiency is the cause of most cysts.

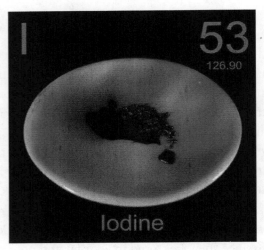

True allergy to iodine is very rare. If you are one of those individuals, then obviously, any form of iodine described below should be avoided.

Two present-day authors have written outstanding books on the protean medical benefits of iodine. They are Dr. David Brownstein and Dr. Mark Sircus. I encourage you to read either or both their books to fully educate yourself on the wonders of using iodine as a medicine. The name of Dr. Brownstein's book is *Iodine: Why You Need It, Why You Can't Live without It*. Dr. Sircus's book is entitled *Healing with Iodine: Your Missing Link to Better Health*.

Iodine deficiency is very widespread in the United States and in fact in many parts of the world. Severe iodine deficiency leads to an enlargement of the thyroid gland (which requires more iodine than any other body organ) or goiter. The farther you live from the oceans, the lower the iodine in your soil.

There are areas in the United States with extremely low quantities of iodine in their soil. Due to that, they had very high rates of goiter and were known as the *goiter belt*. This area went from the Rockies to the Great Lakes Basin to Western New York state.

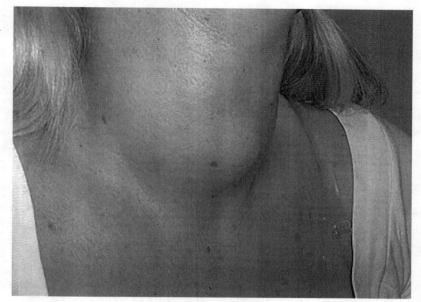

Young woman with early development of goiter (from *Wikipedia*)

After making the far-sighted public health decision to iodize salt, the United States in the 1980s made an abrupt about-face and banned iodine from being added to bread. Iodine was used in commercial bakeries to condition dough, making it easier to bake with.

The totally unfounded fear was that people were getting too much iodine in their diet, which of course was not the case. Incredibly, they chose another halogen named bromine. Bromine, in my opinion, is a poison and, worse, is an antagonist of iodine—meaning that since it has similar properties, it replaces iodine in the body, forming useless thyroid hormones.

The use of chlorine and fluorine in the water supply also wreaked havoc on our bodies, especially our thyroid gland, since they are both similar to bromine in that they mimic the action of iodine. This does not mean that they are capable of replacing the normal activity of iodine in our bodies.

The widespread use of these iodine mimickers, along with lack of iodine supplementation in flour and depleted iodine in our farm soils, produced a perfect storm of iodine deficiency in the United States.

Australia had made similar legislation, but after seeing the iodine levels in their population plummet, they wisely reversed it in 2008. The Australians, like we Americans, were on a low-salt craze and thus even the minimal amounts of iodine they were getting in salt had practically disappeared. Under normal conditions, the salt in your saltshaker loses almost all of its iodine due to evaporation. Plus, if you tried to get your iodine only from salt, you would die due to its toxicity at the high doses you would require.

Bromine wreaks metabolic havoc on the body, and this legislation needs to be reversed immediately. The good news is that when you supplement with iodine, your body will preferentially use it and displace the bromine imposter. In those patients, you will find very high levels of bromine in their urine. Losing bromine is a very good thing.

Iodine is essential for brain development. Every doctor knows that low levels of iodine in pregnancy leads to a very small brain and developmental abnormalities. Those patients are known as *cretins*. Iodine is especially critical to brain development and future intelligence during pregnancy and the first three years of life.

What doctors don't know is the flip side of that: supplementing iodine during pregnancy enhances brain development and results in an increase in IQ of over 20 points on average! There have also been studies that confirm that the average child living in an area with iodine-deficient soil has an approximately 12.45 drop in IQ. If you give iodine supplements to them as they grow, they will recover about 8.7 points of IQ.

Dr. Jorge Flechas has done a lot of work on this and has fascinating lectures that you can find on YouTube. Iodine is completely safe for pregnant women when supplemented correctly, so why is it not given to every pregnant woman?

About a hundred years ago, the United States was the first country in the world that required iodine to be added to all salt. This worked very well to provide enough iodine to the average person to prevent goiter but fell far short of what was needed for good health.

Iodizing salt was very farsighted legislation. What they could not foresee was Americans' wide-scale adoption of a low-salt diet. That along with chemical farming that progressively depleted the soil of all minerals and trace elements including iodine resulted in even further reductions of the average American's intake.

Currently, our levels are dangerously low, and I suspect if it continues, there will be a progressive decline in IQs, which appears to have already begun in Northern Europe, Australia, and the United States. In those countries and many others, there has been a progressive decline in IQs since approximately 1975. Nobody seems to agree as to the cause of this, but it appears it is not genetic, from studying members of the same families.

Studies done in China also confirm the drop in IQs associated with iodine deficiency. That begs the question, what the hell are we doing? Iodine is dirt cheap, readily available, and has nothing but truly beneficial side effects. We now know that it has a very miraculous effect on raising the IQs of children, so why is the government not all over this?

It is clearly in everyone's interest to have a more intelligent citizenry, or is it? Perhaps if you wanted a more docile, dumber population, they would be infinitely easier to control. Just putting the question out there.

Iodine was used extensively in medicine in the past but currently is primarily used as an antiseptic. Even today, in hospitals in the United States, part of the routine for prepping patients for surgery is cleansing off their skin with iodine preparations to sterilize it of all pathogens.

No pathogen—be it a bacterium, virus, fungus, or protozoa—can survive exposure to iodine. Iodine quickly penetrates the cell walls of all microorganisms, rapidly killing them. Iodine kills them so quickly that resistance does not develop. However, sadly, other than its topical uses for sterilization, iodine has been forgotten by modern-day physicians despite its amazing properties.

Antibiotics, on the other hand, only work against bacteria, not fungi or viruses. Antibiotics always lead to resistance. This is proving to be a major problem worldwide, fueling the emergence of multidrug-resistant "superbugs."

These superbugs cannot be killed by any one antibiotic and frequently not even by a "cocktail" of different ones. That is not the case with using iodine, nor will it ever be!

Iodine supports a strong immune system in several ways. It helps purify blood, just as it does when we use it to purify water. Iodine is stored in many tissues of the body, including lymphatics. The lymphatic system drains the body tissues; and here in its lymph nodes, it destroys damaged cells, bacteria, and viruses. Iodine is critical for this to be done.

To prevent and treat coronavirus—and all viral infections, especially colds and flus—iodine is a perfect weapon. Application of iodine to face masks and small amounts on a Q-tip to your nasal passages will go a long way to protect you from respiratory viruses of all types. Using iodine to both prevent and treat flu and COVID-19 has been totally forgotten by modern medicine.

In a fascinating book entitled *Iodine: The Forgotten Weapon Against Influenza Viruses* by David Derry MD, PhD, he writes,

> After the 1918 Influenza Pandemic which killed an estimated 30 million people, governments financed research on the Pandemic's causes. Over 25 years, influenza viruses were isolated and methods for killing them with various agents discovered. Iodine was the most effective agent for killing viruses, especially influenza viruses.
>
> Aerosol iodine was found to kill viruses in sprayed mists, and solutions of iodine were equally effective. In 1945, Burnet and Stone found that putting iodine on mice snouts prevented the mice from being infected with live influenza virus in mists. They suggested that impregnating masks with iodine would help stop viral spread. They also recommended that medical personnel have iodine-aerosol-treated rooms for examination and treatment of highly infected patients.

I currently use nebulized hydrogen peroxide with iodine to treat respiratory tract infections of all types. It is an incredibly useful method that I will delve into more later in this book.

There are many good food sources for iodine. Many come from the ocean where iodine levels are high, including cod, lobster, shrimp, tuna, many saltwater fish and all types of sea vegetables including seaweed dishes such as nori, kombu, wakame, dried seaweed, and even seaweed soup, (that does sound kind of gross, but hey, I have never tried it) cranberries, organic yogurt, milk, potatoes, soy nuts, navy beans, eggs, prunes, and Himalayan pink salt.

DOSAGE OF IODINE

Supplementation with iodine can be done in many forms. Let's take a look at a few:

KELP

One of the best natural organic sources of iodine is a large brown algae/giant seaweed called kelp. Kelp is a tall seaweed that grows in tall "kelp forests" in shallow coastal waters all over the world. It is loaded with iodine and other minerals, vitamins, and trace elements.

Kelp also contains all the essential amino acids your body needs. Kelp has the added advantage of being a food that your body is capable of digesting and easily absorbing. It is also inexpensive and readily available.

There is no set dose of kelp. Kelp can be taken as a tea, tincture, or in capsule form. Capsules usually come in various doses; I would take one that provides 250 mcg of iodine a day. If you are really sick, you can double that for a week or so to give your immune system a much-needed boost.

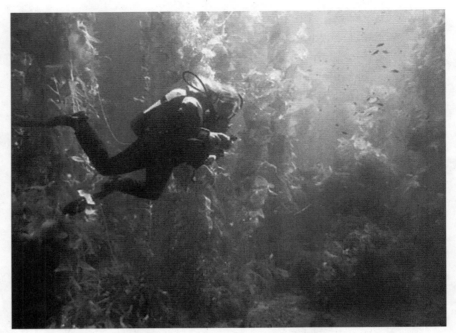

Diver in kelp forest (courtesy of Ed Bierman, Redwood City, USA)

NASCENT IODINE

Nascent iodine is a liquid iodine preparation that is in its atomic form, and thus the most easily absorbed and most readily available form for your body to utilize. It is also the best tolerated form. A few drops can be added to water. I like to rinse it around my mouth before I swallow it since it will also eliminate plaque buildup on your teeth by penetrating the "biofilm" dome, which protects the bacteria in the plaque.

Each drop of nascent iodine contains approximately 0.4 mg of iodine. Since it is soaked up by your mouth directly into your blood, you require less of it. Ten drops a day or 4 mg should provide you with an adequate supply of iodine.

If you get sick, double it for one week then double it again. Don't worry—for the short duration of your sickness, it will not be a problem. The average daily iodine intake among the Japanese is between 13.5 and 45 mg a day due to the amazing amounts of seaweed and seafood in their diet. They ingest these high doses (by Western standards) with absolutely no side effects.

It is also probably why they have one of the lowest rates of breast cancer in the world. The breast is one of the body organs that concentrates iodine in its tissues. That is presumably the reason why iodine deficiency causes the abnormal breast development that leads to breast cysts.

LUGOL'S SOLUTION

Dr. Lugol was a French physician in the 1800s who developed a very potent form of iodine that could be used externally or ingested, without harm. It became a very useful medicine/nutrient for folks to have to treat wounds, skin infections, disinfect water, and taken internally as well. It is an aqueous solution of potassium iodide and iodine.

Lugol's solution was previously sold at 5 percent strength, but the United States government lowered it to 2 percent due to fears of its use in the production of methamphetamines (the infamous crystal meth). The good news is that the 2 percent solution is still very potent and useful for our purposes.

Lugol's solution works very well to treat candida infections and eliminate viruses and other germs from the bloodstream. The dose for an infection such as colds, flu, and the coronavirus is six drops of Lugol's solution mixed with water two to three times a day for the duration of the illness.

Note that prolonged use of Lugol's or any other potent iodine solution does have the potential to suppress thyroid function and should be used cautiously, and it's best to have your thyroid function monitored by your physician (if available and if he or she is knowledgeable about using iodine).

For our purposes, any internal infection would benefit from the addition of Lugol's solution until it is resolved. After which, you can drastically lower its dosage or discontinue it and take iodine in some of the other multitude of forms.

POTASSIUM IODIDE AND IODINE

This combination of iodine and potassium iodide, which is the chemical form of iodine used to iodize salt, is known as Iodoral. It is also used to protect the thyroid gland from radiation by preventing the uptake of radioactive iodine. It comes in 12.5 mg tablets, of which 5 mg are iodine and the rest are potassium iodide. Iodoral is essential to have in case you were exposed to high levels of nuclear fallout/radiation either from an accident at a nuclear plant like the Three Mile Island accident of 1979 or, in the event of the unthinkable, a nuclear war. Wars have the nasty habit of doing what we formerly thought was unthinkable. In fact, isn't that how you go about winning a war? For that reason alone, having some Iodoral on hand could be an invaluable asset. It is very inexpensive and currently readily available. Now is the time to buy some.

Different parts of the body require iodide, such as the thyroid and the skin; whereas the breasts require iodine. If the breasts do not get the iodine they need, they become lumpy and fibrocystic.

Note that for the body to convert iodide to iodine, it needs the mineral selenium. Selenium has wonderful health benefits and is necessary for normal thyroid function. Without selenium, the body cannot convert inactive T4 thyroid hormone to active T3. I will describe the importance of selenium for your immunity shortly.

One 12.5 mg tablet of Iodoral should suffice to provide your body with all the iodine it needs. This is particularly useful if there is a nuclear explosion and radioactive iodine 131 is raining down from the atmosphere. Taking any form of iodine will protect the thyroid gland from taking up radioactive iodine 131, which leads to thyroid cancer.

For more information on the use of Iodoral for radiation exposure, see either of my earlier books, *The Doomsday Book of Medicine* or *The Bible of Alternative Medicine* (both of which are available online at www.doomsdaybookofmedicine.com and www.bibleofalternativemedicine.com).

POVIDONE IODINE SOLUTION (BETADINE)

This is a topical-only solution of 10 percent povidone-iodine mixed in 90 percent water. You cannot ingest this in any form. It still has multiple uses as a topical treatment as well as a disinfectant.

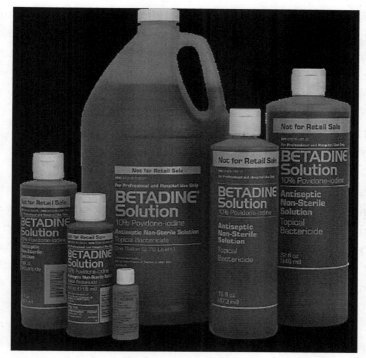

Betadine is fatal to a broad spectrum of germs, including bacteria, fungi, and viruses. It does not burn or sting when applied. It helps to reduce inflammation and is not particularly harmful to healthy tissue.

I strongly advise it for any wound, bite or burn. If left on for some minutes, it will kill all different types of germs, preventing any infection.

You can put some on a Q-tip and clean your outside nostrils after an exposure or as a protective antimicrobial barrier before exposure. If it irritates your nose, dilute a small amount of betadine with equal parts of water and reapply.

SELENIUM

Selenium is a trace mineral that is critical for thyroid function as well as proper immune function, detoxification, and cancer prevention. It is also an essential element in our immune systems arsenal.

Without selenium, the body would not be able to convert inactive thyroid hormone to active thyroid hormone.

As far as an immune function, selenium works along with vitamin E and other antioxidants to soak up and neutralize damaging free radicals. It is also a component of glutathione peroxidase, which protects the cell wall from damage, thus protecting the body's cells.

Selenium also is important in activating your immune system, especially in its antiviral role. Selenium exhibits significant antiviral activity against flu, coronavirus, and other respiratory tract infections. It also inhibits viral mutation, thus preventing potentially more lethal strains of a virus developing in patient's bodies.

That is especially important during a pandemic, as we are currently experiencing with coronavirus. The reality is that all viruses seem to eventually mutate. So far as of the writing of this book, there are twenty-three mutations of COVID-19. There is absolutely no evidence that it is more transmissible or is deadlier for children or anyone else for that matter.

Viruses do not want to kill you. If you die, you are a dead end for them as well, and you cannot continue to spread to new hosts. Viruses want market share that is why they almost always mutate to less lethal forms and even eventually coexisting with us.

Selenium has also shown to be active against bacteria, fungi, and parasites.

Like most vitamins and minerals, selenium is best obtained in foods from which it can be easily assimilated by your body. Foods that are very high in selenium are Brazil nuts. A single Brazil nut contains enough selenium to meet your daily requirement. I personally think four Brazil nuts are the optimal dose.

Other high-selenium foods are tuna, sardines, cottage cheese, mushrooms, and sunflower seeds to name a few. It is also found in significant quantities in brewer's yeast and nutritional yeast.

When using supplements, selenium, like most mineral supplements, is chelated (which means attached) to another molecule, often an amino acid, to facilitate its absorption. You can't lick a rock or suck on stones to get minerals since they are inorganic and, as such, they are not recognized by your body. Your body needs organic material; it has no way to absorb something that is not in organic form.

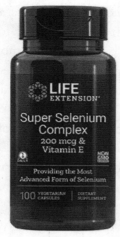

Frequently, selenium is chelated to the essential amino acid methionine, which is then well absorbed by your body. As I mentioned earlier, essential means our bodies cannot manufacture it, so it must be obtained in your diet.

DOSAGE OF SELENIUM

The dose of selenium is 200 mcg once daily with food to further enhance its absorption. In a severe overwhelming infection such as a bad flu, pneumonia, or coronavirus, I would double it only for about ten days max, and then return to your once-a-day dosing to prevent any toxicity. As always, take it with food to help its absorption.

ZINC AND QUERCETIN

Zinc is a mineral that over two hundred enzymes in your body require to properly function. Zinc is also deadly to viruses, which is why over-the-counter cold treatments such as Zicam are so popular.

The Z in Zicam is for its zinc content, and the rest of the name is derived from ICAM-1, which is the receptor that rhinoviruses bind to in order to infect human cells. It is a homeopathic medicine that is not approved by the FDA but seems to be popular with patients.

I have always used zinc to help fight off respiratory tract infections such as colds, the flu, pneumonia, and coronaviruses. It really has no significant side effects, especially for short-term use. Zinc also functions as an antioxidant, although the mechanism for that is not clear.

Zinc also works great for sores in your mouth (aphthous ulcers) and for acne and eczema. Zinc is essential for healing of skin and mucosa such as the lining of your mouth. Zinc is also used in hospitals for patients who recently had surgery and burn patients, in both of which it promotes healing and accelerates their recovery.

I always included zinc in my COVID-19 treatment protocol. President Trump's task force for the coronavirus also recommended zinc as part of their protocol, along with chloroquine and hydroxychloroquine and Zithromax (an antibiotic).

The reason both chloroquine and hydroxychloroquine work against COVID-19 is they act as ionophores, or transport molecules whereby positively charged zinc is shielded and can cross the cell membrane.

The cell membrane has a positive charge, and this normally repels the zinc, preventing its entrance into the cell (since like charges repel each other) and blocking viral replication. Hydroxychloroquine and chloroquine shield the zinc's positive charge and act as a carrier molecule transporting it into the cell.

Thus the use of a zinc ionophore allows zinc to enter directly into the cell and work its magic.

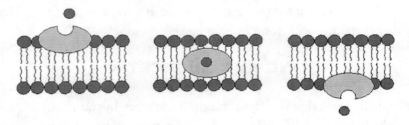

Zinc in red being carried across a cell membrane by the ionophore in green (compliments of *Wikipedia*).

Fortunately for us, hydroxychloroquine and chloroquine are not the only zinc ionophores that we know of. There are natural ionophores that we can obtain without a prescription and are readily available. One of them is quercetin.

Quercetin is a natural pigment found in many of the foods we eat, such as berries, tomatoes, apples, onions, gingko, peppers, red wine, green tea, and even broccoli. It is a flavonoid antioxidant, which is a pigment that imparts color to the foods that contain it.

Quercetin is also available in capsules as a supplement. It is often combined with bromelain to help increase its absorption or combined with EGCG, which is found in green tea. It is also available combined with zinc.

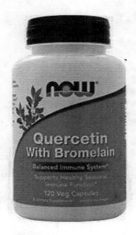

Zinc is known to support and boost immunity, decrease inflammation and, as such, is essential in any plan to treat an infection, especially these viral respiratory infections.

Zinc is responsible for normal development of the immune systems B and T cells, macrophage activity, and modulating uncontrolled cytokine production (which is often fatal).

Studies have shown that zinc will prevent the reproduction of coronavirus in your throat and nasopharynx (the area where the back of your nose and your throat meet). *Therefore* it is very likely that it will also prevent the production of other respiratory viruses that infect the same area.

Cold-EEZE lozenges contain zinc gluconate and will serve this purpose and are easy to find, but any zinc lozenge will suffice. Each lozenge contains 13.3 mg of zinc gluconate. For any of the respiratory infections we are discussing, I would take five or six a day and suck on them slowly, allowing them to dissolve and linger in your throat to interfere with viral replication. Zinc lozenges of any kind will work great to get rid of all ulcers and canker sores in your mouth.

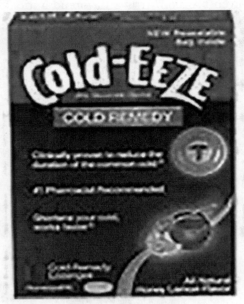

Sucking on zinc lozenges several times a day during any cold, flu, or coronavirus season will certainly help your body fight off this invading viral army.

Zinc is also essential for growth, and deficiencies during childhood will result in stunted growth. It is also responsible for sperm production, testosterone production, and thus, fertility.

Zinc is also involved in protein production as well as DNA production. One odd manifestation of zinc deficiency is loss of sense of smell and taste. Those symptoms are unusual in normal patients.

It has been reported as a symptom of coronavirus, and I wonder if the virus somehow is causing an acute zinc deficiency. Just the ruminations of a doctor from the medical underground Where Doctors in individual practices collaborate and now can share information.

Many of us practice integrative medicine, the combination of both traditional and alternative medicine. As an integrative physician YOU intellectually occupy both worlds, and often wind up with an "out of the box" perspective on things.

If you drill down further on the symptoms of coronavirus, you will find incredibly that many of its symptoms are identical to symptoms of zinc deficiency. Just my own personal observation.

Zinc deficiency is uncommon in the United States since it is contained in many foods. However, I find that despite adequate blood levels of zinc, it always seems to help to supplement it during an infection.

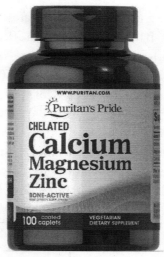

Zinc, like all minerals, must be chelated or attached to a chelating agent such as an amino acid, organic acids, and inorganic acids. This makes the zinc water soluble and easily absorbed by your body.

Common chelating agents added to zinc are amino acids such as aspartate, forming zinc aspartate. Methionine is also used forming zinc methionate. Some organic acids are acetic acid, citric acid, and gluconic acid, making, respectively, zinc acetate, zinc citrate, and zinc gluconate.

Other inorganic acids are sulfates and oxides—forming zinc sulfate and zinc oxide. These inorganic acids chelated to zinc are poorly absorbed, and I would avoid them and stick with the amino acids and organic acids, which have better absorption. It is all about absorption—if you don't absorb it well, then what is the point of taking that form?

Studies have also demonstrated that both niacin (vitamin B3) and selenium help the body absorb zinc. Since zinc is proving to be a central actor in all viral infections, supplementation is key; and once again, absorption is critical. On those grounds, I would suggest supplementing with niacin and selenium along with your zinc. They both have other health benefits with few significant side effects.

Niacin often causes an uncomfortable sensation of warmth flowing through your body known as flushing. Flushing is harmless, just annoying. There are nonflushing niacin preparations on the market, such as niacinamide. Unfortunately, niacinamide is not as active as the flushing niacin's.

The B vitamins need to be taken together as a group—to get your niacin, take a B50 or B100. The B50 has 50 mg of each of the B vitamins, and the B100—yes, you guessed it—has 100 mg of each of the B vitamins. Take one B complex, either B50 or B100, along with selenium 200 mcg along with whatever form of zinc you want to use. Remember, the B vitamins, like vitamin C, are water soluble and as such can be taken on an empty stomach.

Foods that are naturally high in zinc include oysters, red meat, lamb, pork, and turkey. Cashew nuts, sesame seeds, pumpkin seeds, and whole-grain cereals are good sources of zinc. Seafood such as crabs, lobster, shrimp and scallops; dark green leafy veggies; lentils; beans; oats; and yogurt all provide significant amounts of zinc.

DOSAGE OF ZINC

The dose of zinc for the purpose of warding off a nasty cold, flu, or coronavirus is 50 mg a day, until it is resolved. As with all minerals, I would advise taking them with food to help absorb them better. If you are using lozenges, then five or six times a day. Suck them slowly; don't bite them or crush them. Taking zinc for longer than a few weeks must be supplemented with 1 mg of *copper*, since zinc will cause a copper deficiency.

VITAMIN A

Vitamin A is also known as retinol, retinal, and retinoic acid, and includes the provitamin A substances known as the carotenes.

A provitamin is a substance with little vitamin activity until it is converted into a vitamin. Beta-carotene is what gives carrots their orange color. Beta-carotene is transformed by enzymes into retinol or vitamin A. As one would expect retinol is six times stronger than beta-carotene.

Beta-carotene is the most potent of all the carotene family of pigments. The reason is that it contains two retinyl groups that, once broken apart, form two molecules of vitamin A. There are two other carotenes that are active as well but only contain one retinyl group, therefore have half or less the activity of beta-carotene.

Vitamin A is essential for fetal growth and proper development, immunity, and for your vision. It is also responsible for the assimilation of minerals from our diet.

Who among us does not remember their mothers extolling us to eat our carrots they are good for "your eyes"?

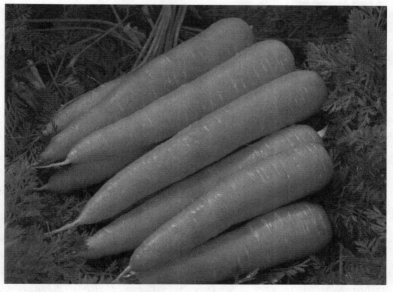

Photo courtesy of Government of Australia Agriculture Dept.

My mother, Mary, was an early reader of *Prevention* magazine in the sixties and was well ahead of her time when it came to nutrition. Looking back, she was amazingly accurate in her nutrition advice, except for her wholesale adoption of margarine instead of butter. In her defense, that was the battle cry of the day.

Now we know that that was a horrific mistake, loading our bodies with fake food loaded with trans fats instead of good healthy fats. Overall, although Mom was a factory worker with no nutritional education, she was self-taught and did an incredible job of feeding us nutritious food on a very thin budget.

Vegetables are not the primary source of vitamin A in most cultures around the world. They mostly get their vitamin A via organ meats such as liver from both animals and fish, butter from cows openly grazed on grass, as well as cream, cheese, and other dairy products. There was also lard and other wonderful sources of healthy fat. They are all jam-packed full of vitamins A, D, and K2.

The vitamins A, D, and K2 act synergistically (work together) to activate your immune system, strengthen your entire body, build strong bones and teeth, and help children grow into tall, strong adults. No one has done more work on this subject than Dr. Weston A. Price.

He was a dentist who traveled the world studying the facial development of primitive tribes. He noted the wonderful facial and physical development of primitive peoples who had not yet adapted a Western diet, and what happened to those who did.

Those "primitive" diets all had one thing in common. They all ate large quantities of animal fats either from fish or land animals. All these fats were jam-packed with the fat-soluble vitamins that are so essential to our health—vitamins A, D, E, and K. The work of Dr. Price is still carried on and can be found at www.westonaprice.org. It is a wonderful organization, part of what I like to refer to as *the medical underground,* since their theories are not accepted by conventional medicine.

Sally Fallon Morell also has written several wonderful and informative books on the principles of Dr. Price that I highly recommend. *Nourishing Fats: Why We Need Animal Fats for Health and Happiness* is one of her latest and is jam-packed full of useful information.

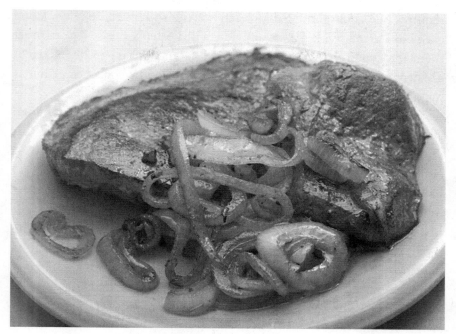

Photo courtesy of CDKitchen.com

Liver, as it turns out, is a nutrient powerhouse, jam-packed full of good fats, minerals, trace elements, and protein.

The reason animal foods such as buttermilk, lard, bacon, cheeses, fish, liver, and others are better sources of vitamin A than plants is that they already contain it and do not require conversion. Plant sources of vitamin A such as beta-carotene need to be enzymatically converted by our bodies, whereas animal sources contain the whole vitamin in a readily available form.

In fact, the animal sources of all fat-soluble vitamins are far superior to any plant sources. This includes vitamins A, D, E, and K. Our bodies assimilate these vitamins from animal sources much easier, thus they are biologically more active and better for us. This is also why whole-food sources of vitamins are far superior to synthetic sources. The only exception seems to be vitamin C, in whose case, all sources seem to have equivalent activity, just vastly differing percentages of absorption.

The FDA allows food manufacturers to list carotenes as vitamin A, which is deceptive. Carotenes need to be converted, and this process requires bile acids and fat-dissolving enzymes (lipases), so if you don't eat your carrots with fat, your body will be hard-pressed to convert them into vitamin A since fats cause bile and lipases to be excreted. This conversion process is also adversely affected by conditions such as hypothyroidism, diabetes, and zinc deficiencies.

Children also have a hard time converting plant-derived foods to vitamin A; hence a low-fat diet is horrific for everyone's health, but especially for pregnant women, infants, and growing children. For your children to grow tall and strong with broad shoulders, strong bones, and handsome, wide, uncrowded faces with beautiful broad smiles, you need to include large amounts of animal fats in their diet, and yours as well.

There has been fascinating recent research demonstrating that the jaws and facial muscles in present-day children are underdeveloped due to a diet of soft processed food. As it turns out, the chewing of fibrous vegetables, often raw, along with meat and fish, is what we were designed for and as such, it leads to proper jaw, teeth, and facial symmetry and development.

A soft, processed modern diet leads to a pinched, narrow face with resulting crowded teeth and ultimately to shrinking, receding sagging jaws and chins. It is making our kids ugly with crooked teeth and weak pigeon-like faces—it is unnatural, and we are doing it to ourselves! Once again, the "old ways" of eating are clearly preferable to our appropriately named SAD (Standard American Diet). Anyone interested in this subject should read the outstanding book describing this common problem, *Jaws: The Story of a Hidden Epidemic.*

Choose grass-fed, organic animals or fish from arctic waters that are not polluted. The reason why grass-fed is superior is that the grasses contain vitamins that are absorbed by the cows in direct proportion to their presence in the grass and then in turn concentrated in their fat. Fish from unpolluted waters are preferable because unlike other fish, they have not concentrated toxins such as mercury into their fat.

However, I digress. Let's get back to why we need vitamin A for a healthy immune system.

Vitamin A helps your immunity in many ways. First and foremost, it is a powerful antioxidant, thus helping to both defend and strengthen our bodies. Studies from around the world confirm that when vitamin

A–rich foods such as liver, cream, butter, and egg yolks were given to children, they were much more resistant to infections.

A deficiency of vitamin A makes you susceptible to infections of all types. Measles seems to be devastating and even fatal in the absence of adequate vitamin A. Vitamin A is used to treat measles and is very effective.

The World Health Organization, or WHO, recommends initially treating infants less than one year of age with 100,000 international units of liquid vitamin A and those children older than one year of age with 200,000 international units.

If the children show any other signs of vitamin A deficiency such as night blindness, dry eyes, or Bitot's spots (grayish-white deposits on the bulbar conjunctiva adjacent to their cornea), then their doses are to be repeated again in twenty-four hours and again in four weeks.

Vitamin A protects your skin and the mucous membranes in your nose and mouth, promotes cilia activity in your lungs, thus helping to clear them. Vitamin A also helps to activate those T cells that rid our bodies of so many nasty infections, including the respiratory tract infections we are discussing here.

In my humble opinion, one of the greatest benefits of vitamin A is how it works so wonderfully along with its two fat-soluble cousins vitamin D and vitamin K2. Vitamin K2 is essential for vitamins A and D to function properly.

All three of these vitamins are essential for good health, and the body and immune system functions better when it has adequate supplies of all three. These three vitamins work together in beautiful synchrony, conferring innumerable benefits on your body and mind.

Once you know this information, it becomes abundantly clear that many of our chronic illnesses and mental afflictions are due to the lack of these essential fats in our diets. The low-fat diet fad was the worst mistake ever made by both incompetent public health officials and self-serving private companies.

Prior to World War II, pregnant women were advised to take cod liver oil daily and eat liver once a week. All that dietary wisdom has been lost on modern medicine. The right fats, iodine, vitamins A, C, D, and K would make a world of difference to the developing fetus and just about everyone else for that matter. Trace elements are in my opinion also essential for the development of a healthy fetus.

I feel that anything that is circulating in our blood normally is there for a purpose. The body does not do anything by chance or without purpose. If trace elements are there, then they have a function, albeit many of which remain *unknown*. Medicine has not done many studies on these trace elements, only noting syndromes that their deficiency causes, but there are no dietary recommendations.

Liver, of course, has the added benefits of being a nutritional superstar, brimming with vitamins, minerals, and trace elements. Liver is high in protein and low in calories to boot. There is no more nutritious food anywhere. Not that cod liver oil is any lightweight when it comes to nutritional content.

Besides vitamin A, cod liver oil contains vitamins D3, E, and fatty acids that are wonderful for your brain, retinas, and skin such as EPA and DHA. The names are brutally long tongue twisters...okay, you asked for it. DHA is docosahexaenoic acid and EPA is eicosapentaenoic acid, that's why I am using their initials!

Amazingly, every cell in our bodies require both DHA and EPA to maintain healthy cell function. Although both DHA and EPA can be manufactured by our bodies from ALA or alpha-linoleic acid. ALA is a fatty acid precursor found in walnuts, canola oil, and flaxseed. The problem is that the rate of conversion is very low, thus it is easier to get your DHA and EPA from animal sources such as cod liver oil, cold-water fatty fish, or supplements. In those sources, no conversion needs to take place, and they are readily recognized by our bodies and absorbed.

In my clinical practice, I have been seeing patients with dry eyes for years. Most are on medications from their ophthalmologists that seem to barely be keeping it at bay. I put them all on a teaspoon of the lemon-flavored cod liver oil, which is available online; and within a month, they are all amazed at the improvement in their dry eyes (without the use of their former medications).

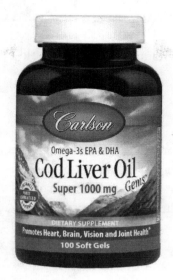

Vitamin A is a powerful arrow in our quiver to use against infections. And like all the other "fat boys" (vitamins D, E, and K) it is an immune-boosting superstar.

VITAMIN A DOSING

As always, the optimal way to get your vitamin A or any nutrient is through whole foods. Foods such as cantaloupe, dairy products, green leafy vegetables such as spinach, liver, and of course carrots.

Cod liver oil and liver of course are the superstars of vitamin A content. One tablespoon of cod liver oil contains about 15,000 IUs (international units) of vitamin A. One serving of liver contains 40,000 IUs of vitamin A.

How much vitamin A should you take it you suspect you have or actually have a bad infection?

I recommend 100,000 international units of non-beta-carotene vitamin A daily for the first four days of your illness. Then if it persists, take it twice a week.

As with all fat-soluble vitamins, there is a potential for toxicity, so you cannot take a high dose for a long time. Remember, it is a fat-soluble vitamin and, as such, needs to be taken with fatty food or you will not absorb it. Remember, any oil is a liquid fat at room temperature, so taking your vitamin A after eating a large salad with olive oil dressing will work just fine.

Note: High doses of vitamins A and D should be avoided by pregnant women.

ASTAXANTHIN

Astaxanthin is a carotenoid similar to carotene, which gives carrots their characteristic orange color. Astaxanthin is also what gives krill and salmon their characteristic pink/red color. Like other carotenoids, astaxanthin is fat soluble, therefore you have to take it with fat to properly absorb it.

Astaxanthin is also found in microalgae, yeast, trout, shrimp, crayfish, crustaceans, and even in the feathers of some birds. Unlike other carotenes, astaxanthin is not a precursor of vitamin A, therefore it does not need to undergo any enzymat.

The primary commercial source of astaxanthin is from a microalga named *Haematococcus pluvial*. This microalga has the highest concentration of astaxanthin found anywhere in nature. Lobsters and crabs are among many other animals that feed on these microalgae and consequently derive their red color from them.

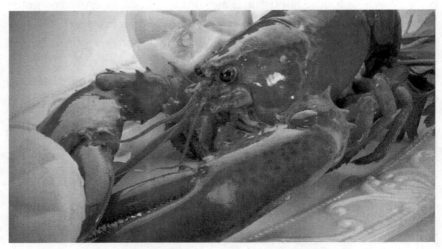

For our purposes, we want to utilize astaxanthin for its powerful antioxidant capacity. As an antioxidant, astaxanthin is 550 times more powerful than vitamin E and an incredible 6,000 times more powerful than vitamin C! As such, it is very useful in the treatment of any infections.

As an added benefit, it also is a powerful anti-inflammatory. It works to interfere with five different inflammatory pathways in our bodies. Reducing inflammation is always a good thing since it is so harmful to our bodies.

DOSE OF ASTAXANTHIN

Currently there are no available dosing guidelines for astaxanthin. Most of the available astaxanthin supplements come in 12 mg doses. If you are sick, I would recommend taking one twice a day with a fatty meal, since it is fat soluble, for the duration of your illness.

If you are using it primarily for prevention, then once a day will suffice.

CHROMIUM

Chromium is a mineral and is considered an essential trace element. It is essential because your body cannot make it, and it is necessary to maintain good health. It is useful in treating patients with diabetes. It is necessary for the production of glucose tolerance factor, which helps the function of insulin, which in turn controls glucose. Chromium is also useful in the treatment of high cholesterol and PCOS or polycystic ovary syndrome. As you know from the iodine section, almost all cysts are a consequence of iodine deficiency.

Chromium has a beneficial effect on the immune system. Chromium helps modulate the immune system, meaning, it "puts the brakes" on when it is overstimulated and conversely, it "hits the gas" when it is sluggish. It helps stimulate the action of B and T lymphocytes, macrophages, and controls cytokine levels.

Foods that are high in chromium include whole grains, beef, poultry, seafood, milk, broccoli, green beans, potatoes, apples, bananas, brewer's yeast, sweet potatoes, molasses, liver, hard cheeses, and even grape juice. You will also be happy to hear the chromium is present in both beer and wine! I have done my part; now, it is up to you to convince your wife that you're drinking beer for your immune health. Good luck with that one.

Note: Chromium should be avoided in pregnant women and those who are breastfeeding. Patients with liver or kidney disease should also avoid chromium supplements.

Chromium supplements come chelated or bound to another molecule. There are about five different types on the market. All chromium is poorly absorbed by our bodies, and among the supplements, the chloride-bound form is the poorest absorbed. Other forms include chromium picolinate, chromium nicotinate, chromium polynicotinate, and chromium histidinate. By far, the most popular on the market is chromium picolinate. It is used in many weight-loss supplements and is the best absorbed of the various chelates.

DOSE OF CHROMIUM

The dose of chromium has not been established. Here, I am not referring to chromium for daily use as a supplement that is in the 50 mcg range. I am referring to using chromium to rapidly boost your immune system. Chromium picolinate, for example, should be 500 mcg capsules. Take two the first seven days then you can lower it to one a day for the duration of your illness.

MUSHROOMS

The environment in which mushrooms grow is a bad-ass neighborhood. In order to survive, mushrooms, over centuries, had to develop methods to ward off the two main gangs after their turf: bacteria and viruses. Hence mushrooms are jam-packed with ingredients that are antibacterial and antiviral.

Penicillin was the first antibiotic discovered, and it is made by a fungus, the *Penicillium* fungi. So for our intents and purposes, we can utilize them to prevent or eradicate infections that are bacterial or viral. Good arrows to have in our quiver. Mushrooms used for health purposes are referred to as medicinal mushrooms.

Note: Do not harvest mushrooms in the wild unless you are very familiar with them and are capable of positively identifying them. There are many mushrooms that appear similar but in fact are a poisonous look-alike. A mistake in identifying a mushroom could easily be fatal!

Medicinal mushrooms produce substances known as beta-glucans, which are complex polysaccharides (chains of sugars, particularly of glucose molecules) similar to starch produced by plants and glycogen produced by animals.

Beta-glucans are known as immune modulators, having properties that stimulate the immune system to fight infections and cancer. Beta-glucans have been shown to both protect against infections and also to shorten their length and severity.

Various types of medicinal mushrooms produce these beta-glucans such as reishi, shiitake, chaga, and maitake. As if that was not good enough, it has also been demonstrated that beta-glucans lower cholesterol levels. But, let's face it, when you have an infection, your cholesterol level is not even among the "top ten" of your concerns!

Beta-glucans have a prominent place in our medicine cabinet in these difficult times since they also have been proven to be effective against anthrax, which is one of the primary diseases used in biological warfare. They also protect the bone marrow from destruction by radiation exposure. After a year like 2020, nothing can be taken off the table as "unlikely" anymore.

Let's take a look at the two most potent of the medicinal mushrooms—reishi and chaga—and their health enhancing benefits. For a more in-depth discussion of the various types of medicinal mushrooms, see either of my earlier two books, *The Doomsday Book of Medicine* and *The Bible of Alternative Medicine*.

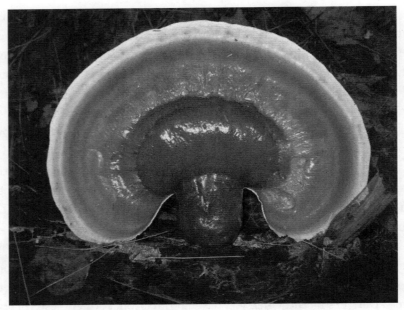

Reishi mushroom compliments of One Green Planet

REISHI (GANODERMA LUCIDUM)

Reishi is a medicinal mushroom that has been used for thousands of years in traditional Chinese medicine. As a medicine, both the mushroom, which is the aboveground fruit of a fungus and the mycelium or underground fungus, are utilized.

Reishi has been used extensively to treat viral infections of the respiratory tract including colds, flu, bronchitis, pneumonia, otitis (ear infections), pharyngitis (throat infections), and sinusitis. Reishi works its magic by boosting the body's production of interferon, which is very potent against viral infections of all types. Reishi also enhances the potency of our body's antioxidants, which is very beneficial overall but especially for infections.

Reishi comes in various colors, but only the red and the black reishi have been shown to have health-enhancing benefits. Wild reishi is another name given for black reishi, which has much less beta-glucan content and hence is not as beneficial as the red.

Avoid raw reishi since it does not undergo the repeated high-pressure boiling that is done to activate the beta-glucans. That process is known as hot-water extraction and is the preferable method for producing potent reishi.

Reishi is usually free of any side effects of any significance, but it may cause some nausea and perhaps a rash. Taking vitamin C at the same time usually reduces side effects by aiding in its rapid absorption. Our old friend vitamin C here once again demonstrating its endless benefits. Drinking lots of water with your reishi also helps it function better as it does for your entire body.

DOSE OF REISHI

There is no set dose of mushrooms such as reishi. Most patients these days take it in the form of a dried extract. Supplements also vary widely in their beta-glucan content, hence making dosing recommendations worthless.

The best way is to carefully read the beta-glucan content on the manufacturers' bottle and use their dosing recommendations. The beta-glucan content is listed as polysaccharides on the supplement bottle labels.

Some people use the mushroom itself, which I would not recommend since as I stated above, there is much less beta-glucan content in the raw unprocessed mushroom.

CHAGA (INONOTUS OBLIQUUS)

Unlike most mushrooms, chaga are not soft but are hard as wood and almost black in color due to its very high melanin content (the same pigment that is responsible for human skin color). Chaga primarily grows on birch trees but occasionally can be found on alder, chestnut, and hornbeam trees. It grows mostly in Siberia and northern Japan but can also be found in the United States as far south as North Carolina.

Chaga is usually found in harsh climates where, in order to survive, it has to produce many different phytochemicals (*phyto* means derived from plants). It is these same phytochemicals that impart many of the health benefits that we associate with chaga and which prompted the Chinese to name it the *king of plants*.

The Siberians, who are no bunch of wimps and are not prone to overstatements, refer to chaga as "the mushroom of immortality" and "a gift from God."

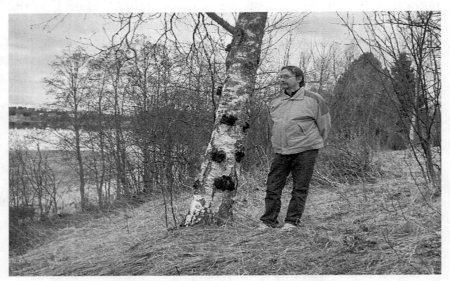

Photo above is of chaga seen growing on a white birch tree; photo compliments of *Wikipedia*.

Chaga contains a large concentration of B vitamins, flavonoids, enzymes, minerals, and phenols—all of which are health enhancing. Chaga is also a potent antioxidant due to its large concentration of the enzyme SOD (superoxide dismutase), which in fact is the highest concentration of it found anywhere in nature. SOD is responsible for breaking down dangerous superoxide anions into oxygen and hydrogen peroxide, hence its beneficial effects on our bodies.

The extraction of these potent phytonutrients from chaga needs to be done before our bodies can utilize them. The phytonutrients are encased in a chitin wall for which humans lack the necessary enzymes and cannot digest them. The most common extraction method is to ground up chaga and make it into a tea.

Chaga's phytochemicals are both water soluble and fat soluble. Making a tea helps extract the water-soluble phytochemicals; the fat-soluble ones need to be extracted using an alcohol such as ethanol. Ethanol is the same alcohol that is used in alcoholic beverages.

Sometimes chaga is fermented, but this is complicated and produces variable results.

DOSE OF CHAGA

Just like reishi, chaga comes in various forms, and there is no set dosage. Chaga is available in beverage form, emulsified drops, syrup, supplements, and tea. As with reishi, look on the label of chaga supplements for either their polysaccharide content or their beta-glucan content, which is the same thing. Try to get a supplement with the highest level of either one.

ENHANCING YOUR MICROBIOME

Even though I have placed this last on our list of ways to boost our immune system, it is by no means the least important. As a matter of fact, most recent research shows just the opposite. It now appears that infections from bacteria, viruses, and fungal sources infect us by a two-step process. The first and most important step is to defeat the good bacteria that inhabit our bodies and keep us in good health. The second step is to overcome the other parts of our immune system.

Let's define what I mean by the term *microbiome*. The human microbiome is all of the different types of microorganisms—such as bacteria, viruses, and fungi—that live on the surface and inside of our bodies. They live in harmony with our bodies. Without them, we could not exist. The cells of the microbiome outnumber the cells of our body anywhere from three to one to as high as ten to one!

The beneficial microorganisms of our microbiome inhabit our skin, conjunctiva (the inside of our eyelids and the surface of the white of our eyes), gastrointestinal tract from our mouth to our anus, urethra, bladder, vagina, placenta, uterus, lung, and even the biliary tract. Many of these areas were previously considered sterile.

The National Institutes of Health or NIH began what is called the Human Microbiome Project in 2007 in an attempt to determine what species makes up our human microbiome and how do they influence our health. By 2012, they estimated that there were over ten thousand different microbial species that inhabit the human body, and the list continues to grow.

There are large numbers of different types of bacteria and fungi and even viruses that coexist in our bodies, each occupying a specific area. Even within the mouth, different species like their own areas to flourish. They work to enhance our immunity by their presence in an area.

Once they colonize an area, that is their turf. Any type of germ, like any invader, has to defeat the locals before they can occupy an area. The microbiome also competes for nutrients with potential invaders in a "scorched earth" system, where they use up the nutrients locally available, thus depriving invaders of food.

There is also an amazing amount of "chatter" going on between the gut microbiome and the immune system. They regulate and support one another. The importance of this communication between the good gut microbiome and the immune system is highlighted by the fact that between 70 and 80 percent of the immune cells of our bodies are located in the gut.

The communication between the gut immune cells and the microbiome is a two-way street. The gut immune cells help the microbiome grow and flourish, and the microbiome send signals to the body that help direct the immune system and fine-tune it to the tasks at hand. It is a symbiotic (mutually beneficial) relationship that, if properly done, results in good gut and overall health and a flourishing community of microorganisms living happily in your gut.

BOOSTING YOUR MICROBIOME

Nurturing your microbiome is probably one of the best things you can do to boost your immunity since it acts as your body's first line of defense and notifies your immune system of the type of attack taking place.

Most of the microbiome inhabits inaccessible areas of your body. There is not much you can do to enhance the microbiome of your vagina, urethra, or even skin. However, you can enhance your gut flora directly by your diet. Since the vast majority of your immune system is related to your gut microbiome, any improvement there will be magnified throughout your body.

A diet that is dominated by plant-derived foods such as fruits and vegetables is a great place to begin. As I mentioned earlier, organic foods are ideal since they do not contain the toxins, pesticides, herbicides, fungicides, and chemical-laden fertilizers. All those chemicals act as poisons on the healthy gut microbiome. In addition to poisoning them, you are also depriving them of the good plant fibers they need to use as prebiotics for food.

The chatter between the gut microbiome and the immune system is via chemical substances secreted by the good bacteria in your gut. Those chemical signals are responsible for informing the immune system about the situation at any given time in the gut. When these chemical signals are disrupted by bad pathogenic bacteria or by toxins or by any other disrupter of the gut microbiome, it is the start of the defeat of the immune system.

When the bad, disease-causing bacteria start to flourish, it throws the gut microbiome out of balance in what is called dysbiosis. Dysbiosis damages the gut lining, causing it to leak, which in turn leads to chronic inflammation, autoimmune conditions, allergies, and disease. That is why it is so critical for your health to maintain a vibrant gut microbiome.

GOOD FOODS FOR YOUR GUT MICROBIOME:

1. Apple cider vinegar
2. Bone broth
3. Fermented foods including sauerkraut, kimchi, kefir, yogurt, fermented vegetables, pickles, miso, natto, and kombucha.
4. Garlic
5. Onions
6. Pineapple
7. Nuts
8. Fiber-rich fruit and vegetables
9. Bananas
10. Mangoes
11. Coconut
12. Wild Salmon
13. Beans

14. Honey (preferably raw)
15. Broccoli
16. Spinach
17. Dandelion
18. Chicory root
19. Asparagus
20. Ancient grains
21. Strawberries
22. Every kind of berry
23. I saved the best two for last: Red Wine and/or dark chocolate

FOODS THAT DAMAGE THE GUT MICROBIOME:

High-sugar foods
Hard liquor
Processed, man-made foods
Trans fats and hydrogenated fats
Refined vegetable oils such as corn, canola, sunflower, soybean, and safflower.
Artificial sweeteners such as aspartame, sucralose, and saccharin
Red meat
Gluten
Fried foods
Farmed fish

CHAPTER SIX

TREATMENT OF RESPIRATORY TRACT INFECTIONS

In chapter 5, I taught you how to boost your immune system in order to make your body as impervious as possible to any infection. That being said, life does get in the way, and perhaps you were not as diligent as you could have been. Many factors potentially can interfere with your immunity, such as stress, depression, sleep deprivation, dehydration, medications, and even coinfections. Whatever the reason, you may now find yourself in the position of having to treat an infection that is just beginning, or a full-blown infection.

The first thing I would do before anything else is to make sure you get a good-night's sleep, especially the first couple days of this new infection. Infections are very stressful on your body, and consequently you will feel exhausted as your body heralds all the resources available to defeat this new invader. I cannot tell you how many times I have felt exhausted and went to bed early and slept for ten hours and woke up feeling back to my old self.

The second thing I would immediately do is to make sure I am well hydrated. Adequate hydration is critical to the proper functioning of your entire body. In addition to which there is a good chance you have a fever, which causes massive water loss across your skin. This water loss is oftentimes imperceptible (you are unaware of it) but can become quite considerate over the course of a few days.

Make sure you drink enough water that you are not thirsty at all and also, more importantly, that your tongue looks wet when you look at it in the mirror. If you look in the mirror and you have a dry cat's tongue, then you need to rapidly ramp up your water intake. Nothing replaces fresh water for hydration.

I can't tell you how many times patients have told me they are hydrating with coffee or non-herbal teas, both of which are caffeinated. Caffeine is a diuretic (it makes you urinate), which will result in worsening of your dehydration.

At the same time, I would ramp up whatever you are currently doing to boost your immune system. Try to double up on your vitamins, minerals, and nutrients that you are currently taking.

If you are not doing anything currently to boost your immunity, I would immediately start on the following five substances to jump-start your immunity and get you on the right track to fight off this infection. Those five substances are the following:

Vitamin C
Vitamin D
Zinc
Iodine
Selenium

That is a good place to start; refer to chapter 5 for the proper dosing of each one. That regimen will jump-start your immune system and will provide it with some essential ingredients in order to fight off an infection. It is by no means the complete list, but you have to start somewhere, and these are all critical components toward that goal. You can pick and choose others from that chapter at your discretion.

Now, you are starting off well rested, well hydrated, and you are providing your immune system with the fuel it needs to start kick starting it into action.

WHAT KIND OF RESPIRATORY TRACT INFECTION DO I HAVE?

Your symptoms will usually direct you to where you are infected. Sometimes it is very easy; the problem is localized to your ears, sinuses, throat, or lungs. By that I mean you have an earache, sinus congestion, sore throat, or cough, which pretty much identifies where the problem lies.

Other times, the symptoms are generalized such as fever, general lethargy, myalgias (muscle aches), arthralgias (joint aches), or just general exhaustion. Often there are combinations of symptoms, fever, headache, sore throat, runny nose, muscle aches, and cough.

Now in the age of COVID-19, there are an entirely new set of symptoms. Symptoms such as loss of taste and or smell are pretty much characteristic of COVID-19, but not always. Some people get COVID-19 and do not have loss of taste and/or smell. I have had a few patients just recently present with several weeks of terrible diarrhea, fever, and generalized exhaustion.

Dyspnea or shortness of breath is a strong sign of COVID-19, but also could just as easily be from a bad bronchitis or a full-blown pneumonia. Other patients present with eye infections such as conjunctivitis. Others present with confusion and neurological signs such as severe headache. Some present with rashes and vascular skin lesions on their toes, the so-called COVID toes. Most present with fever, cough, and fatigue, which is so general it is not helpful in directing us to the proper diagnosis.

As difficult a challenge it may be to properly diagnose what kind of infection you have, it is not that important. "What?" you gasp in outrage. "How could that be?" The reason is for the most part, we will do the same things in order to defeat wherever we are infected. For example, resting and hydrating yourself and boosting your immune system has no downside and will help with any kind of infection you may be carrying.

Let's take a tour of possible respiratory infection sites and discuss how to properly treat each one:

SINUS INFECTION

Your head has several sets of sinuses connected to your nasal passages. The purpose of these sinus cavities is to warm and humidify air before it travels deeper into your body on its way to your lungs. It is also the first spot your body has to begin its defense against possible invaders.

Here are the most common symptoms of a sinus infection:

1. *Headache.* Especially if your nose is not running and your sinus passages are blocked up, the pressure will build in your head. Typically, this pressure feels like it is behind your eyes, sometimes in the cheeks of your face. Sometimes, your upper teeth will become very sensitive, and you might even mistake it for a toothache. Sinus headaches are easy to distinguish from migraines because they are usually on both *sides of your head, and light does not bother you (as it does with a* migraine). An even more important sign is that when you bend over, your headache will become much worse. It will feel like your brains are pushing against the inside of your head, and it will often times throb.

2. *Facial pain and/or swelling.* You may have soft tissue swelling of your periorbital (around your eyes) area or cheeks of your face. These areas will be very tender to touch.

3. *Runny nose.* Usually, once this starts, it will relieve the headache by releasing the built-up mucus. The nature of this mucus will also help us to tell the difference between a viral infection (clear or white mucus) and a bacterial infection (dark-yellow/light-green or dark-green mucus).

4. *Fever.* May or may not be present.

5. *Postnasal drip.* As your sinuses drain, they can go forward out the front of your nose or backward down the back wall of your nasal pharynx or posteriorly into your oral pharynx and then down your throat. You will have the sensation of constantly having to "clear your throat." What you are doing in this instance is hacking up the mucus that has slid down the back of your throat from your infected sinus cavities.

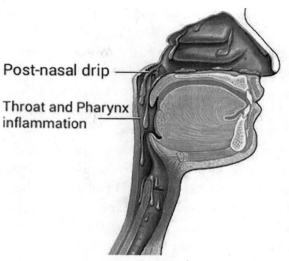

Post-nasal drip

Throat and Pharynx
inflammation

Drawing is compliments of *Wikipedia*.

HOW TO TREAT A SINUS INFECTION

Headaches. Sinus headaches are a totally different beast than migraine headaches. To treat a sinus infection, you need to open up the sinus passages to allow the pressure to be released, which in turn will alleviate the headache. This can be done in several ways. The easiest way is to blow your nose repeatedly to attempt to clear them out. This usually doesn't work, but it might.

Next, you can use a nasal decongestant spray such as Flonase, Nasonex, Nasacort, and Afrin to name a few. They typically work by shrinking the nasal passages, thus allowing the sinuses to drain and relieving the pressure in your head. In my opinion, Afrin by far works the best to open up your sinuses.

However, it is the worst with causing rebound. Rebound means that after a week or so, it will not work for very long, and the nasal mucosa (lining of your nasal passages) will reswell rapidly, nullifying any effect. Saline spray works well, and I like to use that since it does not lead to any rebound effect.

Another very popular way is to use a neti pot—or recently, a new device known as Navage works very well—to flush out your sinus passages. They typically use a saline solution to irrigate your nasal passages and sinuses.

The formula for the saline solution if you need to make it is a teaspoon of salt and a pinch of baking soda in two cups of water. You can use your neti pot as often as you like, but typically, three or four times a day does the trick. The neti pots are passive and use gravity to flush out your nose. Navage is battery operated and uses suction to pull the mucus out of your nasal passages. It comes down to personal preference.

I personally like cold or ice packs to relieve sinus headaches. I keep a couple of ice packs in my freezer for when I feel a headache coming on. The ice or cold packs will cause the nasal and sinus lining to shrink from the cold, and this will oftentimes relieve the obstruction and hence the headache. I also immediately take two Excedrin tablets for the pain.

Excedrin is a combination of caffeine, Tylenol, and aspirin and works very well for sinus headaches. I also take an antihistamine at the same time to help shrink my nasal passages and thus relieve the pressure. If it is nighttime, I will take Benadryl, which is sedating and will help you get back to sleep. Zyrtec can also be used; if so, I would recommend giving it at bedtime since it may be sedating.

If it is during the day, I suggest using a nonsedating antihistamine such as Claritin or Allegra. If you have the decongestant with it such as Claritin-D or Allegra-D, even better, but they occasionally require a prescription. I usually use two ice packs; I apply one to the back of the neck and the other across my forehead.

Usually, if I take the medications and apply the ice packs, I can sleep for an hour or even less and get up and feel better. When I do arise after wiping out the headache that a half hour before was killing me, I typically like to exuberantly yell to my wife, "The kid is back!" Of course, my wife, Lynne, being who she is, loves to reply, "Honey, I think the 'you being the kid' ship has sailed." Alas, she might be right. However, I digress.

You can use a variety of analgesics (painkillers) to treat the pain of the sinus headache, but nothing works better than relieving the obstruction by the above methods. If you need an analgesic, your choice typically is

Aleve (naproxen)
Advil or Motrin (ibuprofen)
Tylenol (acetaminophen)
Excedrin (Tylenol, aspirin, and caffeine).

Note: Aspirin should not be used for pain relief due to its potential to irritate the stomach and possibly cause a GI bleed. Aspirin also has an adverse effect on your platelets and hence should be avoided.

You should take Aleve, Advil, or Motrin with food since they can irritate your stomach. Excedrin should be taken with food, but typically is rather well tolerated. Tylenol does not cause GI upset and can be taken on an empty stomach with no problem.

Another tried-and-true method of relieving obstructed sinuses and hence a headache is to use steam. Place a bath towel over your head to trap the steam and put your face over your sink and run the hot water full blast. Inhale the steam through your nose, not your mouth; this will loosen the impacted mucus obstructing your sinus and melt it away, thus allowing the mucus to escape and relieve the sinus obstruction.

Be careful to keep your eyes closed during this since the steam may irritate them. You can add a little Vicks to this to help decongest and open up your sinus passages. Vicks makes its own steam machine for this that you can find online.

Facial pain and/or swelling. Many of the above treatments for headache will also work to reduce facial swelling. Ice packs are the best for doing this quickly and effectively. Antihistamines, nasal sprays, neti pots, and Navage will also work to open up clogged sinus passages and thus reduce facial swelling. I would be careful using steam to relieve your facial swelling, since it may cause more swelling of your sinuses in the short term, making your discomfort worse.

Runny nose or rhinitis as it is known medically. The antihistamines work very well to dry out a runny nose. Afrin and the other nasal sprays mentioned above also work very well. Saline spray or even a homemade saline solution will also dry out your nasal passages. Steam will also do the trick. Decongestants such as Mucinex will also help this.

In the Far East, they oftentimes will chew on a clove of ginger to dry out a runny nose. Hot tea with honey is also used to dry out a runny nose.

Avoid smoking since smoke is an irritant to your nasal passage, and often, your body will react to this by pouring out fluid in order to wash away the offensive irritant.

Fever. Fever should not be treated unless it goes up very high, above 102 in an adult. Even then, I would be reluctant to treat it unless the patient was very uncomfortable. The reason, as I mentioned earlier in this book, is that fever is one of your body's great defenses against infection.

The bugs that infect us can only do so because they live at our body temperature. Your body attempts to kill them off by cooking them alive with a fever, making their present living arrangements very inhospitable. Hence do not treat a fever unless you have no other choice; you are working against yourself, and it will only work to prolong your illness.

Postnasal drip. This is treated in the same way as a runny nose since all it is essentially is a runny nose in the opposite direction: down your throat instead of out your nose.

NEBULIZATION: THE MOST EFFECTIVE METHOD TO TREAT ALL RESPIRATORY TRACT INFECTIONS

Nebulization is a method of delivery of substances via a machine called a nebulizer. A nebulizer has a small cup inside of it, which contains the medicinal liquid (such as hydrogen peroxide) that you want to use. This small cup of liquid is connected to a compressor by a tube inside the nebulizer.

The compressor forces air into the tubing that vaporizes the liquid in the cup. This produces a smokelike mist of microscopic bubbles containing the medication. These bubbles are able to penetrate all the way from your nasal passages and sinuses into your pharynx and larynx and then through your bronchi to the deepest recesses of your lungs.

Hence it becomes a wonderful tool for delivering medication to otherwise unreachable areas of your body. Via nebulization, you are able to treat nasal and sinus infections, throat infections, bronchitis, and even pneumonia.

Originally, these small home nebulizing machines were used exclusively to treat asthma. Patients were able to deliver asthma medications like albuterol at home without having to make a visit to the doctor's office. It is extremely useful in treating patients who are in intensive care units and also for infants who cannot swallow medication.

Now these home nebulizers are very inexpensive and readily available online or in pharmacies without a doctor's prescription. I would definitely recommend buying one now and learning how to mix the medications and use it properly. Do not buy the handheld models; the compressors are too weak, and therefore the machines are not powerful enough.

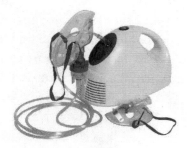

For decades, all over the world, doctors have used hydrogen peroxide to treat infections, especially viral infections where our options are quite limited. Remember, antibiotics only work on bacterial infections, not viral or fungal ones. It was originally given intravenously; then some enterprising doctors began using it via nebulization with outstanding results.

Hydrogen peroxide has the chemical formula H_2O_2. It consists of a water molecule (H_2O) and an extra oxygen atom (O). When it is metabolized or broken down inside the body, it forms water and a single-oxygen atom. That oxygen atom is deadly to viruses and bacteria. It causes them to fall apart, killing them on contact.

Hydrogen peroxide is produced naturally by your body and is contained both inside the cells and in the spaces around the cells. It is what your immune cells concentrate inside of them to be released upon contact with infected cells or microorganisms, such as viruses, to kill them. It is incredibly effective in this role. Part of its beauty is that it is so lethal for invaders but harmless inside of your body once it breaks down into oxygen and water.

Nature once again has come up with a simple formula of two harmless substances that, when combined, are lethal to viruses but with little collateral damage from its release inside of the body's tissues.

Hydrogen peroxide is readily available in grocery stores, pharmacies, and even convenience stores. It usually comes in a dark-brown plastic bottle and is a 3 percent concentration. This form of hydrogen peroxide is fine for the short term.

However, this form does contain chemical stabilizers in it, which very likely are inert and not a problem. But if you "have concerns" about stabilizers, then get food-grade hydrogen peroxide. Recently, there is 3 percent food-grade hydrogen peroxide. Food-grade often comes in much higher concentrations, such as 12, 18, and 35 percent.

Recently online, it has become difficult to find the 35 percent, which is not a problem; the 12 or 18 percent mixes are easier because you don't need to dilute them as much to achieve your desired dilution level.

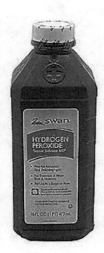

There is a wide range of medical doctors (as opposed to PhD's with degrees in the history of lesbian dance) who are now utilizing these treatments in their offices. They are using it in various dilutions. Some utilize the full 3 percent strength; others dilute it in half or a third to 1 percent. Others dilute it even more to a fraction of 1 percent. There is no right or wrong here; all the various dilutions work down to a tenth of a percent.

However, sometimes, there is a little bit of stinging and irritation to the nose and airways from the full 3 percent strength. I think 1 percent is easy to dilute and maintains a significant amount of its potency, with little to no stinging and irritation.

To achieve such strengths, you will need to dilute your hydrogen peroxide. You should use saline to dilute the peroxide since plain water, with its lack of electrolytes in it, may potentially damage your lung tissue. If you are desperate, you can add a pinch of salt to sterile water and use that.

Don't freak out if your magic potion is a little bit off; there is more than enough room for variability in the potency without sacrificing efficacy. To make your own saline mix, the easiest formula is to take a cup of water and add half a teaspoon of salt. Table salt or sea salt will work just fine.

Note: Be very careful handling 35 percent hydrogen peroxide. It is very powerful and will cause a chemical burn on you. NEVER EVER USE THIS STRENGTH ANYWHERE IN OR ON YOUR BODY. IT MUST BE HEAVILY DILUTED BEFORE IT BECOMES HARMLESS. DO NOT EVEN LET IT TOUCH YOUR SKIN.

HERE IS A QUICK DILUTION GUIDE:

For 35 percent hydrogen peroxide: to get a one percent solution, mix one part of the hydrogen peroxide with to thirty-four parts of saline.
For 18 percent hydrogen peroxide: to get to a 1 percent solution, mix one part of the hydrogen peroxide to seventeen parts of saline.
For 12 percent hydrogen peroxide: to get a 1 percent solution, mix one part of the hydrogen peroxide with eleven parts of saline.

When I say *one part* in the above formula, that can be any size you want. One drop, one cup, one ounce, one quart—you pick it. If you want to mix your peroxide ahead of time and store it, you should pick a cool, dark place. This will slow any breakdown of your mix.

Now, as if that wasn't good enough—wait, there is more! As you recall from the last chapter, iodine is a very potent germ killer to all types of pathogens, and especially to viruses. Putting iodine on the snouts of mice and exposing them to flu and other viruses gave them near-total protection.

Iodine also has the added advantage of causing your immune systems killers—the white blood cells—to increase their content of hydrogen peroxide! Thus adding a single drop of iodine to your nebulizer solution makes it a much more potent mix.

As you recall, there are various mixtures of iodine. For nebulizer use, the two that are safe to use internally are Lugol's solution and nascent iodine. They both are super potent. My personal preference is nascent, but it is much more expensive. Either one will work just fine.

Most pharmacies carry Lugol's solution, but not nascent. Naturally, both are available online. If you have premixed your nebulizer solution, do not add the iodine. Wait until you fill up the dispenser cup inside the nebulizer and then add a drop of either type of iodine right before you use it.

Getting back to the nebulizer—many come with only a mouthpiece. That is okay if you are just using it for your lungs. However, I prefer to use the face masks, which you can buy separately and are relatively inexpensive. I would buy several of them. If you have children you want to treat, then buy the children's-size face mask since the adult size will be much too large and therefore ineffective due to leaking.

You can do these nebulizer treatments at any interval you find effective. Initially, if you are very sick, you may want to do a treatment every two hours. Once you start feeling better, you can move that up to every four or six hours.

When using the nebulizer, sit in a comfortable position, put the mask on (make sure it is snug to your face but not uncomfortable). Inhale slowly and deeply. This will allow the solution to coat your nasal passages and sinuses and work its way deep into the far recesses of your lungs.

You don't have to necessarily wait until you are sick to use your nebulizer. If you feel you had a significant exposure to someone who is ill with COVID-19, flu, or other respiratory tract infection, you can take a treatment once or twice a day for several days just to eradicate any potential invaders.

Besides using hydrogen peroxide in your nebulizer, you can use magnesium. You can use magnesium either as magnesium chloride or magnesium sulfate (Epsom salts) or magnesium oil.

Epsom salts is available in any pharmacy and most grocery stores. Magnesium oil and magnesium chloride are available online. The easiest and most readily available is Epsom salts.

Mix approximately one-third of a teaspoon of Epsom salts in a teaspoon of water and put it into your nebulizer. You can use several of these same mixtures if you need to fill your nebulizer cup.

Don't be overly concerned about getting a third of a teaspoon of Epsom salts; the ratio is not that critical. You can use this as often as you like, the same as the hydrogen peroxide mixture.

Since it is a salt, the Epsom salts may crystalize in your tubing. That is no problem; just flush it out with warm water. Those same crystals may also potentially block the air hole from the compressor in your nebulizer—once again, easily remedied by flushing it out with water.

For the magnesium chloride, mix 7.5 grams of magnesium chloride or 3.5 teaspoons of magnesium oil into 100 ml of water. This will make a large batch of it. Just store it for later use and shake it well each time to make sure it is adequately mixed.

I cannot stress enough the critical importance of buying a nebulizer with all the supplies you need now and becoming comfortable with using it. In the likely outbreak of another pandemic or a biological warfare attack, you will not be able to find a nebulizer machine, tubing, masks for you and your children and even food-grade hydrogen peroxide or iodine solutions. *Now is the time to buy the entire set* of supplies for your nebulizer.

EAR INFECTION

The ear is comprised of three parts. There is the external auditory canal, which is the tube-shaped structure that connects the outer ear to tympanic membrane (the eardrum). This is the part you clean with a Q-tip.

Hopefully, you don't go any deeper and perforate (put a hole in) your eardrum. Many patients have large, perforated eardrums; and for them, it is possible to go into the middle ear through the hole in the damaged eardrum.

Naturally, the eardrum and the external auditory canal are involved in hearing. If the external auditory canal is blocked with wax or a pustular discharge, it will cause a muffling in your hearing. That is a sure sign something is wrong with your ear. It might just be wax or some dirt, but often, it is the early sign of an ear infection.

Fluid in the middle ear will also muffle one's hearing. A discharge of pus in the external auditory canal is a sign of an external ear infection or swimmer's ear since this is the kind of ear infection folks most often get from swimming in contaminated lake or pond water.

Some patients get it from swimming and not drying their ears well. Not usually a problem in the ocean with salt water. If you pull on the ear itself and it hurts, that is a sign of swimmer's ear. The external canal may be red and inflamed, possibly itchy or not, may or may not have a warm discharge of pus, usually not foul smelling.

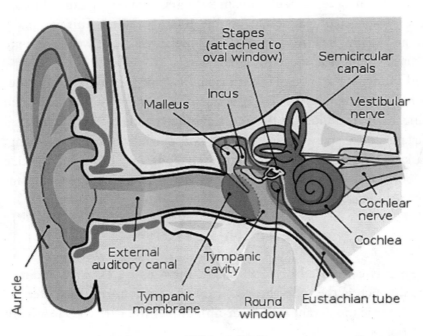

Courtesy of Wikimedia Commons.

The drawing above shows the middle ear in pink and the Eustachian tube that drains it. It is a quite-thin tube and can easily get blocked. The middle ear is also involved in hearing, and any problem with it will affect your hearing.

Ear infections usually do not begin with an earache; that usually takes a few days to build up. One of the first signs is a feeling of pressure in your ears. This may alternate between ears, be a single ear, or involve both ears.

Many times, you will notice sinus pressure and maybe the start of a headache that feels like it is "behind your eyes." Upper respiratory tract infections typically include the ear, sinuses, and throat or any combination thereof. Now, let's get back to the ear.

A middle-ear infection will include ear pain, sometimes very sensitive to even a light touch. The pain may be deep inside the ear or in front of the ear, the area between your sideburns and your ear. Other times, it may involve the side of your head behind your ear. The pain may be mild to severe in nature. Many times, there will be vertigo (dizziness) and even nausea. A middle-ear infection may or may not include a fever. If it does, remember to "let it burn."

The most common ear infections involve the middle ear followed by the outer ear, and a very distant last place goes to inner-ear infections.

The third part is the inner ear—infections here will make you dizzy. Hence diminished hearing and/or dizziness will be your first signs of an ear infection. Once you know the anatomy, you can really understand how the symptoms develop. You will often have ringing in your ears, hearing loss, and balance problems when you are standing or walking. The room may spin, and you may get nauseous and experience vomiting.

HOW TO TREAT EAR INFECTIONS

Unlike the other parts of the respiratory tract, the ears are very inaccessible to us. We can reach the outer ear up to the eardrum. We also can open up the middle ear by opening the Eustachian tube. Unlike the rest of the respiratory tract, we cannot reach any part of the ear with nebulizer treatments.

Let's take a look at how to treat the various kinds of ear infections.

Swimmer's ear or otitis externa. The first thing you need to do is to clean all the debris out of your external ear canal. Be very gentle when you are doing this since the infected outer ear will be tender to any touch.

Take a turkey baster with its rubber ball on the end, or an infant's ball syringe, and fill it with a mixture of half warm water and half hydrogen peroxide. Have the patient lie with their head down on a bed with the painful ear side up. Insert the tip of the turkey baster into your outer ear canal and gently and repeatedly flush out your ear until the water coming out is clean of any debris. Do not use very hot or cold water; both may cause a very painful reaction from your pissed-off ear.

If you don't have a turkey baster or infant's ball syringe, then just lay the patient down and pour the hydrogen peroxide–warm water mix directly into the ear, filling it up. Allow it to sit there for several minutes and then have them turn their head and drain it out. Do this repeatedly until the outer ear canal is clean.

Instead of the hydrogen peroxide, you can substitute it with white vinegar, either undiluted or diluted, with sterile water in a 50-50 mixture. Another mixture you can use is half rubbing alcohol and half whiter vinegar.

You can also use a mix of mullein and garlic in oil. Here is the recipe for that potion:

Take four or five cloves of garlic, crush them, and mix them in a pan and allow to sit for fifteen minutes. Then add a quarter cup of dried mullein. Now get the "virgins," either one ounce of EVOO (extra virgin olive oil) or virgin coconut oil, or mix the two if you like. As you may recall from earlier in this book, they both have antiviral properties.

Place your mix into a small saucepan inside a larger one that is half full of water. Heat it until the water is warm, without cooking the garlic. Now take it and strain it through a coffee filter or cheesecloth to remove all the particles of garlic and mullein.

At this point, you can either use it as is, or you can make it even more potent by the addition of several drops of a carrier oil, which will allow it to penetrate deeper. You can use either tea tree oil, oregano oil, lavender oil, or eucalyptus oil. Use two or three drops of this up to six times a day.

Heat is a mainstay of treatment for a swimmer's ear infection. You can use a heating pad or microwave a facecloth or small towel. Lie with the painful ear down onto the source of your heat. Do this for fifteen minutes or so several times a day. Heat helps to soothe your ear infection and helps open up a clogged ear and allow it to drain, which in turn relieves a lot of symptoms.

An old-time remedy for an outer ear infection, which I thought was pretty ingenious, was to use an onion. Leaving the skin on a large onion, bake it for fifteen minutes to twenty minutes then cut it in half. Allow it to cool just a little so you don't burn your ear and apply the cut half to your ear and hold it in place with a towel. This will transmit both warmth and moisture into your outer ear, soothing it and helping it to possibly open and drain.

Note: Do not flush out your ears or use any eardrops if you have a perforated eardrum or if you have myringotomy tubes (ear tubes) in place.

Taking a cotton ball and soaking it in peroxide and placing it inside the outer or external auditory canal will also help to treat a swimmer's ear infection. You can leave it in there for hours, changing it several times a day.

A very potent disinfectant for the outer ear is iodine. It is preferable to use a water-based iodine such as Betadine, Lugol's solution, and nascent iodine rather than an alcohol-based iodine. The reason being if there is a perforation of the ear drum, alcohol-based iodine may damage the inner ear.

You can either soak a cotton ball in a few drops of Lugol's or nascent iodine and insert it into the outer ear canal and rotate it gently so in effect, you are wiping the canal walls. Or you can put a few drops of any of the three water-based iodines in some warm water or hydrogen peroxide. Iodine mixed with peroxide is a very potent mix against all pathogens.

I would do this twice a day until the ear feels better. You'll know when swimmer's ear is healed when you no longer have any ear discomfort even when gently tugging on your ear or pressing against the underside of it, as if to fold your earlobe over your ear opening.

The pain from an outer ear infection can be treated with over-the-counter analgesics such as Tylenol, Advil, Aleve, Motrin, and ibuprofen. A very potent combination for pain relief includes Tylenol or acetaminophen and either Advil, Motrin, or ibuprofen.

Take two of each with a large glass of water, preferably on a full stomach. Studies have shown that this is as potent as a narcotic analgesic. As mentioned earlier, heat will also help the pain; occasionally, ice packs will help—everyone's reaction is different.

Middle ear or otitis media infections are treated in a different fashion. Since we don't have direct access to the middle or inner ear, our options are much limited.

Once again, heat from a heating pad or moist hot towel will help open up and drain your middle ear. Fluid collecting in a middle ear from a collapsed Eustachian tube is the cause of most of the symptoms from a middle-ear infection. A variation of this is to use steam. You can boil a large pot of water, remove it from the heat, and make a tent over your head with a large bath towel. This will trap the steam under the towel and you can inhale it thru your mouth. Do this for several minutes, several times a day if needed.

Use the painkillers as described above for the outer-ear infection.

Antihistamines and decongestants will also help with the fluid buildup and also with any dizziness or vertigo. You can use Sudafed, Benadryl, Claritin, Allegra, Zyrtec, or Xyzal.

Over-the-counter nasal sprays will also help open up your Eustachian tube, such as Nasonex, Nasacort, Afrin, and Flonase. Spray them up each nostril, snort them in deeply into your nasal passages, wait five minutes, and then blow your nose and repeat it.

Your primary goal here is to open a blocked Eustachian tube. If you have ever flown and had ear problems, that is your Eustachian tube closing on you from the changing air pressures in the airplane. Some ways to open it include yawning repeatedly or chewing gum.

Another tried-and-true method is the Valsalva maneuver. To perform this, you pinch your nostrils closed, open your mouth, and take in a mouthful of air and forcibly blow it out through your nose. You will often hear your ears give a small pop. Do this repeatedly.

A different method is known as the Toynbee maneuver. This is similar to the Valsalva maneuver. You pinch your nostrils closed with your fingers, and with them closed, you drink a glass of water.

Saline nasal spray will also help relieve an obstructed Eustachian tube. Take the nasal spray and direct it deeply into your nose. Fill up your nose canal and then snort it deeply into your nasal passages by pinching the opposite side and drawing air into your nose.

Another method is to instill warm water mixed with peroxide into your outer ear and leaving it in there for ten minutes by lying on your good side and keeping the bad ear up. You can also use warm olive oil for the same effect.

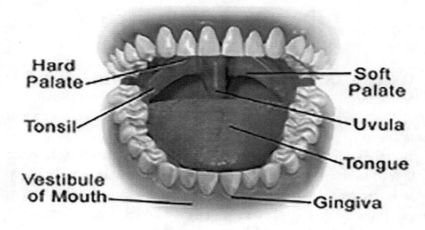

Mouth

Compliments of *Wikipedia*.

THROAT INFECTIONS

Pharyngitis or throat infections are relatively straightforward to diagnose: you have a sore, scratchy throat. It becomes painful and difficult to swallow, sometimes even to talk. Your voice may become hoarse and weak. This sore throat may or may not be accompanied by swollen glands in your neck that may also be painful to touch.

If you look into the throat, there may be patches of pus on the back of the throat or on your tonsils. If you still have your tonsils, they are easy to spot. They lie on either side of the very back of your mouth; they look like little pink balls, about the size of a small bean. If they are infected with a bacterium, they will likely have a pustular discharge leaking from their surface. This is referred to medically as tonsillitis.

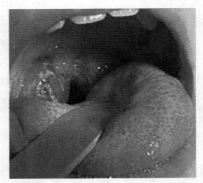

Tonsillitis compliments of *Wikipedia*.

Colds, flu, COVID-19, respiratory viruses, and bacteria such as streptococcus all cause throat infections. Viral infections usually are self-limited, meaning they burn themselves out—in this case, in about a week or so.

Bacterial infections could be serious, especially strep throat, which could lead to damage of multiple organs from rheumatic fever. Strep throat is frequently accompanied by other symptoms such as high fever, fatigue, muscle aches, swollen painful lymph nodes in your neck, and a generalized "feeling like crap" known as malaise.

HOW TO TREAT THROAT INFECTIONS

The wonderful thing about throat infections is the excellent access we have to the throat to treat them. We have a variety of topical treatments we can utilize that are extremely effective. Let's take a look at various treatments.

When using any of the following solutions for a mouth rinse and gargle, you should allow the mixture to fill up the back of your throat and gargle for a few seconds followed by a swishing of it between your teeth and around your mouth; then spit it out.

Iodine and water. You can put several drops of iodine in a small glass of water and gargle with this mixture every four to six hours. You can use Betadine, nascent iodine, or Lugol's solution. Just like on the skin, iodine is a very potent antimicrobial. It is still used in medical settings all over the world to sterilize surfaces and instruments. The reason we still use it is that it is so deadly to germs that there is little chance to develop resistance.

Hydrogen peroxide and water. Fill half a small glass with hydrogen peroxide and the rest with water. Use this solution every four to six hours.

Baking soda or salt. Use half a teaspoon of either one in a small glass of water and use that mix every four hours. Spit it out when you are done.

Apple cider vinegar. Do not use this undiluted. As you can imagine, pouring vinegar in a raw throat will be very uncomfortable to say the least. One or two teaspoons of apple cider vinegar in a small glass of water will do. Gargle with this mix every four to six hours, but if it helps you can do it as much as you want.

Nebulized hydrogen peroxide. Using a nebulized mixture of hydrogen peroxide and water is a very effective treatment for throat infections. The directions are spelled out earlier in this chapter. You can do this every four to six hours, or more often if you need to.

You can also soothe your throat with hot tea and honey. Chamomile tea is an old favorite for this. Hot chicken soup also works to soothe your throat and also boost your immune system.

The Irish recommend adding a little whiskey to your tea and honey to give it some extra punch. The honey helps promote healing, and the whiskey just takes your mind off the whole mess! You have to love the Irish.

Strep throat usually needs to be treated with antibiotics and you should see a doctor if your throat pain persists, especially if it has a pustular discharge. A tonsillitis or infection of your tonsils themselves will sometimes require surgical removal.

Zinc lozenges also work great to soothe and heal any mouth sores from any cause. Aphthous ulcers, also known as canker sores, are small painful sores, oftentimes with a white or gray color to their center. They may occur on the mouth, lips, or tongue.

They may be alone or with a few of their buddies scattered around your mouth. I have been curing this 100 percent of the time for over three decades by using zinc lozenges. They are caused by a zinc deficiency, not an infection.

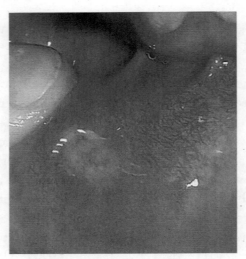

Compliments of *Wikipedia*.

The mineral zinc is required for all wound healing, but especially the lining of the mouth known as the mucosa. Zinc lozenges are readily available either online or from your local pharmacy. Use your tongue to hold the lozenge directly over the canker sore until it dissolves. Use these lozenges four or five times a day until they are healed.

LUNG INFECTIONS: BRONCHITIS AND PNEUMONIA

An infection of the large airways or bronchial tubes leading to the lungs is known as bronchitis. Once the infection reaches the air sacs or alveoli in the lungs, it is known as pneumonia. For our intents and purposes, we will treat both types of infections the same way. However, you should be aware that pneumonia is more serious and can often be fatal, especially in young children and the elderly.

The classic symptom of either bronchitis or pneumonia is a cough. Coughs are distinguished by if they produce phlegm or mucus (which is a wet cough), or nothing is coughed up (which is a dry cough). If your cough is wet, the next thing to analyze is its color. Viral infections typically produce sputum (phlegm or mucus), which is clear or white.

Bacterial infections typically produce purulent sputum, meaning it is yellow, green, or brown in color. Although yellow sputum, sometimes if light in color, may be caused by a viral infection. If sputum is laced with streaks of red or is rusty colored, this is a bad sign, indicating blood admixed with your sputum. Rusty sputum should be evaluated by a doctor as soon as possible.

Other symptoms of bronchitis and pneumonia include shortness of breath. This is especially prevalent in pneumonia but can be present in both. Chest pain also occurs and is usually made worse by coughing, laughing, and deep inspiration. Often the chest wall itself will be tender to touch, and this is from inflammation of the ribs and their attached cartilage. That condition is known as costochondritis. It frequently takes weeks to even months to completely resolve. Generalized muscle aches known as myalgias are often present.

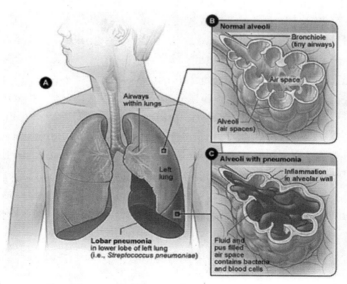

Compliments of National Institutes of Health.

Fever and shaking chills known as rigors are often symptoms of lower respiratory tract infections, especially pneumonia and COVID-19. Rigors are usually accompanied by a rapid rise in body temperature.

Extreme fatigue often accompanies these infections and will last beyond the resolution of the infection, until the body fully recuperates. It takes a lot of energy and resources for your body to fight a serious infection such as pneumonia. The result is exhaustion. Dehydration almost always occurs from fever, sweating, and fluid loss from excess sputum production. That is why I always recommend rest and hydration as the first steps in treating any respiratory tract infection.

Sometimes, these infections have symptoms outside of the respiratory tract such as nausea, vomiting, and diarrhea.

In cases where the oxygen levels drop too low, especially in the elderly, there will be accompanying confusion. Low oxygen levels also can produce cyanosis, which is a bluish discoloration of the skin, lips, or nail beds of fingers. Either confusion or cyanosis is a very bad sign, and those patients will need medical attention as soon as possible. These patients need supplemental oxygen immediately.

COVID-19 produces the same symptoms as above with a few new twists. It oftentimes causes loss of taste and smell. Sometimes, it causes vascular lesions such as discoloration of toes known as COVID toes. COVID-19 also seems to produce a rapid onset of severe shortness of breath and respiratory failure.

It also causes multi-organ failure in susceptible patients that are either elderly or suffer with other comorbidities. Severe diarrhea that lasts for weeks has also been described in COVID-19 patients. It is proving itself quite adept at producing a myriad of different symptoms.

Anyone who has blood in their mucus, high fever (higher than 101.5 degrees F) for more than a week, increasing dyspnea (shortness of breath), persistent lethargy, or persistent chest pain should be evaluated by a physician as soon as possible. These symptoms are all signs of serious complications that may become life-threatening.

HOW TO TREAT BRONCHITIS AND PNEUMONIA

I will start this section with methods in common for treating bronchitis, pneumonia, and the flu. In the next chapter, I will give treatment recommendations that are unique to COVID-19.

As are my recommendations for any infection, you should start with excellent hydration as well as getting a good, minimum eight-hour-a-night sleep. In the case of these lower respiratory tract infections, hydration helps keep the mucus loose and more fluid-like. If you become dehydrated, which is often the case, then your sputum will become thick and jelly-like and more difficult to expectorate (cough up).

Thick mucus causes a repeating hacking cough in an attempt by your body to clear your airways of these thick mucus plugs. The best fluids to hydrate with are water, apple juice, and broth. Do not use coffee or non-herbal tea since they are caffeinated and are diuretics, thus making you lose fluid. Also avoid alcohol, which does not work well for hydration purposes, although it may take your mind off of the pneumonia!

I shouldn't have to state this, but smoking should be avoided when you have a respiratory tract infection. I have learned over decades of being in practice that some people are just idiots, and you have to spell out everything for them. So, even though it should be painfully obvious that smoking is going to make your cough worse, I feel compelled to say it.

If you are not currently taking any immune-boosting supplements, you should start the quick-start program immediately. Refer to chapter 5 for directions on how to start immune boosters from scratch.

If you are currently supplementing, then raise your doses. Vitamins C and D should especially be ramped up. Double your vitamin D, making sure you are taking it with a fatty meal. Double your vitamin C every two days or until you get diarrhea. If that happens, cut back to the previous dose or a lesser dose you can tolerate. If you are taking liposomal vitamin C, you will most likely not have any bowel problems.

Now let's get to the specific treatments for the lower respiratory tract infections of bronchitis, pneumonia, and COVID-19. Due to their relatively inaccessible location deep inside our bodies, treating lung infections has its own set of challenges.

By far, the best method of treating any lung infection is via nebulization. No treatment has a faster onset of action and a lack of adverse side effects as nebulization. I described how to dilute hydrogen peroxide to use in a nebulizer earlier in this chapter under sinus infections.

Never use full-strength hydrogen peroxide—it must be diluted. The addition of a drop of iodine (in any of the forms I described earlier) to the nebulizer solution will make it a much more potent killer to any bacteria or viruses.

There is no steadfast rule as to how often you should use the nebulizer treatments. I would suggest every four hours initially and see how it works. If needed, you can ramp it up to every two hours or even every hour. It has no major adverse side effects, and generally, it is very well tolerated.

As I described earlier in this chapter under sinus infections, you can also use magnesium in your nebulizer treatments. Magnesium helps relax the airways, opening them up, mobilizes secretions, and helps patients with asthma who have exacerbations (flare-ups) from respiratory tract infections.

I described how to use magnesium in its various forms earlier in this chapter. You can dose magnesium just like hydrogen peroxide nebulizer treatments. I would advise four times a day to start, and you can adjust that in either direction, depending upon your response.

Magnesium chloride can also be used to treat infections. Since it has both antibacterial and antiviral properties, it has been used historically to treat infections before the advent of antibiotics. Now in this new age of antibiotic-resistant infections, many of these old treatments are being revisited, especially by integrative physicians such as myself. Dr. Raul Vergini has pioneered its recent usage against infections of all types.

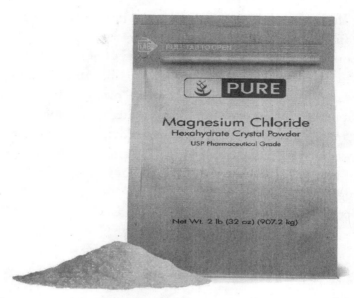

Magnesium chloride can be used via nebulizer as described, but it is also a potent antimicrobial when administered orally. Magnesium also is a bronchodilator, meaning it opens up the airways that lead deep into your lung, allowing you to breathe better. It does this by relaxing the smooth muscle that surrounds the bronchi.

You can mix up a large batch of this to be taken orally. You have to make a 2.5 percent solution, which means 25 grams of magnesium chloride powder mixed in one liter of water. That would be a little under four teaspoons of pure magnesium chloride as in the brand in the photo since it is 6.6 grams per teaspoon.

For adults, give 125 cc every six hours. As they improve, increase the dosing interval to every eight hours, then every twelve hours. Continue every-twelve-hour dosing for several days after they appear to be recovered. For children, use half the dose; and for infants, use 15 cc.

Besides working to kill the bugs that are infecting you, it also helps over three hundred enzymes in your body that require magnesium. Note: only use magnesium chloride in this fashion, not the magnesium oil or the magnesium sulfate.

Iodine can also be nebulized without hydrogen peroxide. Simply put several drops of either 5 percent Lugol's solution or nascent iodine into several cc of saline solution and use the nebulizer like you always would. This is much more potent than the hydrogen peroxide–iodine mix. Iodine kills all pathogens on contact

Steam is also very helpful with these types of infections. You can either stand under your shower and run it very hot and inhale the steam for a few minutes or make a tent with a towel over your head and inhale steam from a pot of water or run the hot water in the sink.

Steam helps break up the thick mucus and helps you bring it up. The hot air will also dilate (expand) your airways, allowing more oxygen in and also facilitating the coughing up and out of sputum from deep in your lungs.

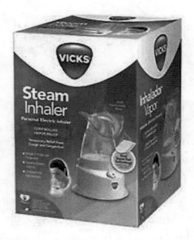

The addition of Vicks or a drop of eucalyptus oil will also help to open up your lungs and aid in decongestion. Vicks makes a small steam inhaler that is relatively inexpensive that will work for our purposes. This will help sinus infections as well; it will break up any impacted mucus in your sinuses and help loosen it. I have fond memories of my mother rubbing Vicks VapoRub on my chest as a child—it worked then, and it works now.

If you have any inhalers such as albuterol (ProAir HFA, Ventolin HFA and AccuNeb) and Xopenex, now is the time to use them to help open up your airways. Use them four times a day until you recover. Coffee and tea are also bronchodilators, albeit weak ones.

Steam and magnesium will both work to open up your airways. Anything that does expand or dilate your airways will allow more air to enter your lungs, making breathing easier. Dilation also facilitates the clearing of copious amounts of purulent sputum from deep in your lungs, unclogging your airways.

As with other respiratory tract infections, there is oftentimes significant head congestion and rhinitis (runny nose). To treat these, nothing works as fast as antihistamines such as Allegra, Benadryl, Claritin, Clarinex, Tavist, Xyzal, and Zyrtec to name a few of the more popular ones.

If they have a D designation after their name, then even better since this stands for decongestant. They are all nonsedating, except for Benadryl and mildly sedating Zyrtec. Intranasal (nose) sprays such as Afrin work very nicely as well—but remember, it causes rebound, so do not use it for more than one week. Flonase, Rhinocort, Nasacort, and Nasonex do not cause rebound but are not as strong as Afrin.

You can also use guaifenesin or Mucinex in its various forms for both decongestion, cough suppression, and as an expectorant to help "bring up" sputum so you can clear your lungs. It is very effective at cough suppression and clearing of mucus from your airways. It is available without a prescription.

Mucinex D is guaifenesin and pseudoephedrine, which is Sudafed, a nasal decongestant. Sudafed works by shrinking the blood vessels in the nose, thus drying out the nasal passages. Mucinex DM is guaifenesin and dextromethorphan, an effective cough suppressant.

Now let's take a look at several natural medicines that will help fight off viral and bacterial infections. Some are directly virucidal, others bactericidal, some are both and also stimulate your immune system.

The list of herbs and other treatments that follows gives you a selection from which to choose from. Certainly, I am not implying that you need to take all of these. This simply gives you a list from which to choose what you think you need at any given time.

Echinacea and goldenseal. Echinacea's botanical name is Echinacea purpurea; its common name is coneflower. It is widely available in capsule form to be used medicinally. It is also widely planted in American gardens including my own for its beauty. Goldenseal's botanical name is *Hydrastis canadensis*—try to say that three times after a few drinks!

These two herbs work synergistically, meaning they enhance each other's health benefits, each working to stimulate different parts of our immune systems. Echinacea also has antiviral properties and is thought to reduce both the length and the severity of a viral illness.

Goldenseal has been used for centuries by American Indian tribes, especially the Cherokee. The potency of goldenseal is derived from several alkaloids it contains, which include berberine, hydrastine, and canadine—all three of which have astringent properties, meaning they dry out mucous membranes and thus eliminate runny nose and sinus and head congestion. In addition, goldenseal has both anti-inflammatory and antimicrobial effects (meaning it kills all types of germs).

Fortunately for our needs, various companies have these two wonderful herbs combined in one capsule. Some have the addition of cayenne, burdock, and garlic among other herbs. All of which is supportive of your immune system. The doses of the two main ingredients varies among the different manufacturers but is usually in the 400 to 500 mg range.

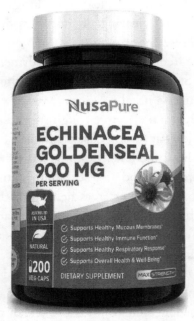

Another very popular supplement for respiratory tract infections is elderberry (*Sambucus nigra*). Elderberry grows wild in much of the Unites States and is also grown as a popular garden shrub for its delicious berries. I am a big fan of it and have several stands of it growing on my farm, despite the ceaseless efforts of local white-tailed deer who seem to crave it as much as I do.

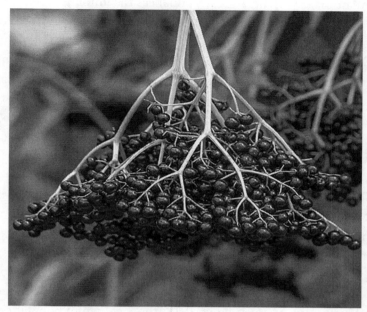

Elderberry is popular for good reason—it works very well due to its various beneficial effects on our bodies. Some of which include a strong antiviral and antibacterial effect as well as an anti-inflammatory effect. By the way, any anti-inflammatory effect is helpful to cure many different illnesses since inflammation does so much damage to our health.

Elderberry is commonly used in cooked form as a syrup, juice, tea, tincture, or tonic. You cannot eat uncooked elderberries since they may cause gastrointestinal upset with resulting diarrhea, nausea and even vomiting. It is also available in capsule form in various doses. Elderberry should not be used by pregnant or nursing women.

Another powerful herbal treatment for respiratory tract infections is *Andrographis paniculata*. It is also called Kan Jang and is often referred to as "the king of bitters" due to its bitter taste. It is used extensively in Ayurveda and traditional Chinese medicine to treat colds and respiratory tract infections of all kinds. For over a decade, it has been the most popular cold remedy in all of Scandinavia.

The active ingredient in andrographis is known as andrographolide. Andrographolide has several health-enhancing benefits. It is a strong anti-inflammatory agent, it greatly enhances the immune system, lowers blood pressure and blood glucose levels, protects the liver from toxins, and inhibits the production of blood clots, which is particularly useful in COVID-19 since it causes vascular problems and blood clotting.

Andrographis comes in various doses, usually 120 mg, 300 mg, and 400 mg, depending on the manufacturer. Take it four times a day until your infection is resolved.

Note: DO NOT USE THIS IF YOU ARE PREGNANT SINCE IT CAN CAUSE MISCARRIAGES AND TERMINATE YOUR PREGNANCY.

Lomatium dissectum is another amazing botanical that has been described as the strongest native antiviral plant in existence. It is in the carrot family and grows in the Pacific Northwest. Its common name is fernleaf biscuitroot and has been used by the local native tribes for centuries.

It always amazed me how indigenous peoples were able to find medicinal plants such as this, but alas, they did and it worked great for them. During the Spanish flu of 1918, the local white population was devastated, but the native tribes used *Lomatium* and fared quite well. In addition to being antiviral, it is also antifungal and works quite well against *Candida albicans* infections.

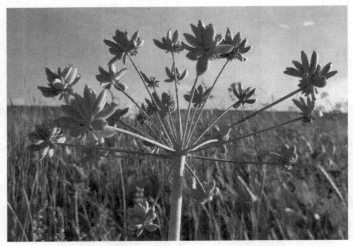

Lomatium dissectum photo by Thayne Tuason.

Candida lives normally on your skin, mouth, throat, gut, and vagina. Sometimes, it grows outside of the gut and other areas and leads to systemic fungal infections. In fact, *Candida* is the most common fungal infection in the United States.

Another strain of *Candida*, known as *Candida auris*, has recently emerged in health-care facilities in the United States and is proving to be multidrug resistant and therefore quite dangerous. This highlights the importance of having an antifungal treatment that is potent and readily available without a prescription and without the side effects that prescription medications often have.

Lomatium is available in various forms such as a tincture, tea, and capsules. The doses are as follows:

Tincture. Take 2 to 4 ml four times a day. You can also mix the tincture in a cup of hot water. Mix a quarter of a teaspoon in a cup of hot water and drink it every four hours for about five days.

Tea. Take one or two teaspoons of the dried herb and pour a cup of boiling water over it. Allow it to steep for twenty minutes or so and then drain off the tea. Drink this three times a day until the infection is resolved.

Capsules. The capsules usually come in 900 mg doses. Take two capsules daily with a meal to help increase its absorption.

Note: *Lomatium* may cause a whole body rash that is red and raised. The good news is that it will disappear without any residual problems once you discontinue it.

I like to use a combination of the andrographis and the *Lomatium* together as a one-two punch against respiratory tract infections. This combination will supercharge your immunity while at the same time acting as a very potent antiviral.

Now, let's take a look at some cough syrups we can use. As I mentioned earlier in this chapter, Mucinex is a very effective cough suppressant as well as an expectorant. Other things that soothe an irritated throat will also help with a mild cough, such as tea with honey and lemon and chicken soup.

A cough remedy I really like involves my favorite juice, pineapple. I absolutely love pineapple juice and drink it on a regular basis. Pineapple juice is full of healthful ingredients. It has lots of vitamin C, magnesium, and calcium. The enzyme bromelain is found in the core or stem of a pineapple as well as its juices. Canned pineapple has very little of this wonderful enzyme.

Bromelain is a potent anti-inflammatory, and as such, it decreases the inflammation in painful joints and muscles. Thus it relieves the aches and pains you have when you are sick. Since bromelain is a protein-digesting enzyme or protease, it helps with your digestion.

Bromelain even helps with allergies by breaking down the mucus. For the same reason, it also works well as a cough medicine, helping to digest and break down the thick sputum that is sticking to your airway walls.

Here is the recipe for pineapple cough medicine courtesy of the Nourished Life:

One cup of pineapple juice, two tablespoons of honey, a quarter cup of lemon juice, and a pinch of sea salt, and if you like, a pinch of cayenne pepper or ground ginger.

Blend ingredients well and store in a mason or other glass jar in your refrigerator. Take one to three tablespoons as needed to soothe a sore throat, cough, or cold. Adding a splash of Grey Goose vodka might help take your mind off your cough. What the hell—it will help you to relax. Let's face it, you are not going anywhere with this infection. You need to rest; however, I digress.

Honey was one of the ingredients in the pineapple cough medicine, and for good reason. Studies have shown that honey helps suppress coughs and also soothes your throat. And it tastes great. You can also mix in yogurt and eat it if you prefer. The best way is to put two teaspoons in some herbal tea, squeeze some fresh lemons into it, and sip it slowly. Drink a cup three times a day as needed for your cough.

A similar cough syrup can be made using ginger. Ginger is an anti-inflammatory and also works to relax spasmed airways, thus helping a cough in two ways. Take some organic ginger powder, ginger tea, or fresh ginger slices, steep them in hot water. Add honey and lemon juice to make it taste better and to enhance its health benefits.

Another effective treatment for cough is the spice turmeric. Turmeric contains curcumin. Curcumin is excellent for the treatment of respiratory tract infections of any type since it is antiviral, antibacterial, and an anti-inflammatory agent.

Black pepper helps to aid in the absorption of turmeric. BioPerine is a patented formulation of black pepper that is often added to turmeric capsules to help its absorption.

Turmeric often comes as a powder. You can mix one teaspoon of turmeric with 1/8 teaspoon of black pepper. Mix it in either a tea or a cold drink. Turmeric is also available in capsules, many times already formulated with black pepper or BioPerine. The dosage of the capsules varies between 600 mg to 1,500 mg. There is no set dose to take; it should be taken between two and three times a day, depending on the severity of your illness. It works nicely to suppress cough and has been used in Ayurvedic medicine for centuries. It is also sometimes mixed with ginger.

Another common home remedy that works well for coughs include cayenne pepper, ginger, apple cider vinegar, and our old stand-by: honey. You can prepare any quantity of cough medicine you want using this basic ratio of ingredients:

4 parts apple cider vinegar

4 parts honey

1 part cayenne pepper

1 part ginger

Mix this together, put it in a glass jar, and take a sip or two of it as often as you need to suppress your cough. It is a little fiery in taste but will do the trick and stop that cough.

THE INFLUENZA OR FLU

The influenza virus is commonly known as the flu. It is no coincidence that the name sounds like the word *influence*. In Latin and Italian (which is basically street Latin), the word *influentia* means "to influence."

In medieval times, the people were generally very superstitious. They felt that "la infuenza" was caused by a misalignment of the stars of the zodiac and by spells, which naturally have a "bad influence" on folks.

There are four known types of flu viruses: A, B, C, and D. Human influenza types A and B are responsible for the seasonal flu we suffer from every winter. Type A is the only flu virus that has the ability to cause worldwide epidemics, also known as a pandemic.

These pandemic-causing type A flu viruses are only able to spread globally if they are highly contagious and easily spread between people. Type C flu viruses or influenzas usually cause mild disease and do not cause epidemics. Type D influenza only infects cattle and does not spread to humans.

Influenza A is further divided into subtypes according to the two different types of proteins on the virus surface. One of the two surface proteins on influenza A is called hemagglutinin designated by the letter *H*, which has eighteen different subtypes, named H1 to H18.

The other protein is neuraminidase designated by the letter N, which has eleven subtypes, designated N1 thru N11. The naming of the various subtypes of influenza A are therefore designated H1, N1 for example.

These subtypes are the result of mutations in the influenza A genes, resulting in new types of proteins being produced. By nature's natural selection, eventually, there will arise new flu type A viruses that will be much more contagious. Eventually, one of those new mutations is super infectious, and you have a pandemic on your hands.

"How is that natural selection?" you ponder. The less infective viruses will not get the opportunity to multiply and, from the viruses' perspective, will therefore not be as succesful. The only strategy that matters to a virus is one that results in the virus spreading and replicating far and wide.

That is why being fatal is not in its evolutionary interests because a dead person cannot spread the virus to others. In fact, oddly enough, we are now coming to realize that many viruses attach themselves to us permanently by providing an evolutionary trait that increases our survival.

Once a beneficial trait like that is inserted by the virus into our DNA, by natural selection, those people who carry it will have a greater chance to survive and reproduce. Hence it is passed on from generation to generation, and those viral genes become a permanent part of our genome.

Freaky stuff, when you think about it: *we are viral*. Viruses may very well turn out to have "the greatest" influence on human evolution. As I learn more about viruses, the more impressive I find them. We are virtually surrounded by a magnificent world of viruses termed the *virusphere*. There is a wonderful book by Frank Ryan of the same name. If you are a science lover like me, and want to learn more about viruses, you will relish this book.

Influenza B is further divided into two main lineages: B/Yamagata and B/Victoria. There are a large number of subtypes under each lineage. The influenza B viruses are much more stable than the influenza A viruses, thus their surface proteins change slowly, and they don't produce as many novel subtypes as influenza A viruses. Hence from a human standpoint, influenza B viruses are not as much of a threat to us as influenza A viruses.

The reason being there is a very good chance we already have antibodies to its surface proteins. Therefore conferring immunity to us from a perfect match to antigens stored in our immune systems library of earlier infections.

Pretty cool stuff, and you can see why it had to develop; otherwise, we would be susceptible to every infection as if it was new. Once again, our old friend natural selection comes into play. Those with stronger immune systems are conferred with a huge survival advantage. More of them survived each epidemic, and so did their genes.

The virus strains to be included in the annual flu vaccine arise from extensive disease surveillance done by the CDC in Asia every year. The vaccine usually includes two types of influenza A viruses and one or two types of influenza B viruses.

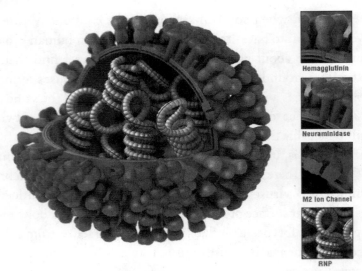

A drawing of influenza A and its surface proteins (CDC).

The flu is a highly contagious virus. Flu patients spew virus into the surrounding air in two forms. Large droplets of water/saliva/sputum in which contain infective flu virus—that is the lesser modality of spread. The most common is via aerosol. Aerosol in this case refers to gases (air) that contain viral particles in suspension.

It is able to travel many feet from an infected person by coughing, sneezing and just plain breathing, the infective distance being determined by the force one breaths out with. Think of blowing a smoke ring—the harder you blow, the farther the smoke goes. Picture that smoke as an aerosol filled with virus, thus you can see how far you are contagious to other people.

Masks only protect you from the large water droplets, not aerosol. If you can breathe through it, so can the virus pass through it. Dr. Fauci telling us that masks will stop viral spread is a total lie. None of our esteemed members of the press asked him the key question: If surgical masks and cloth masks are so effective in stopping viruses, then why are they wearing space suits in the virology labs?

By the way, flu is infective via many routes such as that runny nose of yours, your saliva (spit), your feces, and even your blood. Touching an infected surface infects your hands, and from them it is transmitted to your face—and then you are screwed. That is why handwashing periodically during your busy day is so effective in preventing many respiratory tract infections including the flu.

Once the virus enters your respiratory tract, either via your nose, sinus passages, or mouth, it immediately gets to work. There are specific protrusions on the surface of the cells of those areas; the virus recognizes them and immediately acts like Velcro, attaching itself to the surface of the cells that line our respiratory tract.

It is by no accident these viruses have coevolved with mankind. Flu viruses are perfectly adapted to both live at our exact body temperature and to attach to the surface proteins of the respiratory tract cells it needs to infect in order to gain entry into our bodies.

Once they attach to the outer membranes of these respiratory cells, they trick the cell into opening up its outer envelope, and thus giving the virus entry into the cell and then into the nucleus or control center of the cell. Once in the nucleus, it inserts itself into the operating software of the cell—the genes—and starts reproducing itself.

The virus eventually explodes the cell by producing too many of itself, and thus it spreads to the rest of the body. The immune system only has a small window to put out this fire of an infection before the person gets sick. This is the incubation period. It is only the incubation period if you get sick. If your immune system wins, you will never know it. Which makes perfect sense. Why send a signal that you conquered an invader? It confers no advantage to the person. Your body is superefficient and would never do anything as worthless as that.

The incubation period for the flu is one to four days after exposure, with an average of two days. That is not much time between exposure and getting sick. Patients become contagious at least one day before they know they are sick, spewing virus everywhere they go and onto everyone they come in contact with. A lot of the contact is seemingly as benign as shaking hands or hugging someone.

Flu is further spread by patients who have immune systems that are not strong enough to prevent the infection but are strong enough to never develop symptoms. They feel fine but they are shedding virus, infecting people everywhere they go.

I like to use the analogy of if the common cold is a summer breeze, the flu is a hurricane hitting you. Patients who have the flu typically are sick as dogs. Colds are so named because you typically don't have a fever. Flu, on the other hand, typically causes a high fever of 100–102 degrees F or greater for three or four days. Children tend to run very high fevers from the flu.

Your muscles ache like hell, you are exhausted, you have a dry hacking, horrific cough, while at the same time your head is pounding and feels like it's about to explode. Patients feel exhausted, especially at the onset of the flu. But this fatigue may last for weeks after the flu has resolved. Head congestion and a sore throat may occur but are not typical side effects.

The public, for some odd reason, remains blind to the fact that the flu is one of the most deadly viruses man has faced. Annually, it kills tens of thousands of Americans—ninety thousand plus in a bad year is not unheard of. The Spanish flu of 1918 was one of the most lethal in history, killing between twenty and thirty million people, and a significant factor in causing the end of World War I.

The flu has its favorite victims—the old and enfeebled and the immunocompromised as well as the young and weak. Despite vaccination attempts, hundreds of school-age students die annually, many of whom had severe asthma and allergies. Kids carry the flu and get the flu, unlike with COVID-19, where they do neither.

FLU PREVENTION

As I mentioned earlier, personal hygiene is very important in flu prevention. If you can block the transmission of flu virus from your hands touching your face, that will go a long way in keeping you free of the flu.

Sometimes, the old ways are the best. Long ago, scientists discovered the power of iodine to kill microorganisms of all types. If you knew you were in the middle of a flu pandemic and were probably going to be exposed to it quite often, then using iodine for prevention is quite effective.

If you are wearing a mask, a couple drops of either nascent iodine, Betadine, or Lugol's solution strategically around the mask will make it a virus-killing barrier. You could also put some liquid iodine in any of its forms on a Q-tip and insert it into your nose just about the same distance as the cotton end of the Q-tip.

You don't have to insert it very far at all. If it hurts, you went too far, or you are a complete wimp. With the Q-tip soaked with liquid iodine, slowly swirl it in a complete circle to provide a virus-eradication zone in your nostrils, which are a principal port of entry for flu viruses.

Now let's talk about the effectiveness of the annual flu vaccine, your so-called flu shot. According to the CDC, the annual flu shot varies from 10 to 60 percent effective. It all depends upon two factors, the match between the new infectious mutations and the vaccine, and the person's underlying immunity, vigor, and comorbidities (other diseases).

Flu, in my humble opinion, can easily be prevented by supplementing with vitamin D3 and vitamin C. As I described in chapter 5, sunlight is key in determining when the flu season occurs. The reason is that sunlight striking human skin produces vitamin D.

Since flu is a direct result of a vitamin D deficiency, then one would expect when sunlight is the weakest, flu would be the greatest. That is certainly the case worldwide. Winters with their bad weather and lack of sunlight are exactly when flu season occurs. Many studies have confirmed that the outbreaks of respiratory infections, including the flu, correlate with latitudes, and thus directly with their sun exposure.

Keeping your vitamin D levels between 60 ng/ml and 80 ng/ml, not the standard 30 ng/ml, is much more effective than any flu vaccine. Additionally, vitamin D produces antimicrobial peptides, which act as natural antibiotics in the lung, preventing infections as well as treating them. Vitamin D also helps prevent exacerbations (flare-ups) of asthma, thus also helping respiration.

Vitamin C works synergistically with your immune system, thus its importance in preventing all diseases, including flu viruses. I would therefore recommend taking vitamin D3 between 5,000 and 7,500 international units daily, with a fatty meal to ensure its absorption. That should be more than enough to keep your vitamin D blood levels up to the task of preventing flu and other respiratory tract infections, including COVID-19.

I would recommend 2 grams (2,000 mg) of vitamin C in two divided doses daily. Vitamin C is water soluble and, as such, can be taken on an empty stomach or with a meal; it has no effect on it.

I will talk about the doses I want you to take if you are infected later on in this section.

Rest and a charged-up immune system will go a long way in preventing the flu. What I spoke about earlier—using various antioxidants, minerals such as zinc, mushrooms, probiotics, and other immune boosters—will also help in prevention of any infection, including the flu. Those recommendations are universal for any infection that you may contract.

Zinc is vital in both the prevention and treatment of all viral infections. If taking chelated zinc supplements is not part of your daily supplementation, you should strongly consider adding it. As I mentioned earlier, the zinc supplement you get should be chelated with an amino acid to help vastly increase its absorption. Some of the best forms of chelated zinc to use are zinc aspartate and zinc methionate.

Remember that zinc is much more effective when taken with the plant pigment quercetin. Quercetin is an ionophore, meaning it opens up the cell membrane to allow zinc to enter the cell where it is lethal to viruses. That along with a supercharged immunity will go a long way in both preventing and treating the flu. You can now buy them combined together as a single supplement.

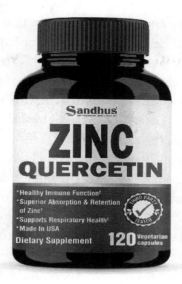

TREATMENT OF THE FLU

Some of the old treatments for the flu, before the current era of antivirals, were indeed reported to be quite effective and have been all but forgotten today.

Baking soda, or sodium bicarbonate, was indeed one of those early ingenious methods of treating respiratory tract infections such as the cold and flu. It exploited a basic vulnerability of all viral infections: their love of an acidic or low pH.

The reason for this is viruses need an acidic environment in the "terrain" of the body. The terrain is the area between cells and around the cells; it is also called the extracellular space, and the fluid in it is known as the interstitial fluid. This area needs to be acidic or the viruses are unable to attach to the cells to gain entry. If they cannot get into the cell, they are unable to reproduce and infect you.

This treatment with baking soda was exploiting the theory of changing the terrain, making it inhospitable to viruses rather than attacking them. At the time, this was the great controversy in medicine—Louis Pasteur theory of germs as the cause of disease called the germ theory vs. the terrain theory of Claude Bernard, which treated the terrain or environment to be what caused disease.

The germ theory eventually was the one that prevailed; however, it was said that on his deathbed, Pasteur recanted and his final words were, "The microbe is nothing, terrain is all." You have to hand it to old Louie; he came clean just in time! I personally think that fully embracing germ theory and totally denying the terrain theory was a monumental mistake. Let's take a look at what happened when the terrain was changed in the treatment of the flu.

During the deadly Spanish flu of 1918, doctors used sodium bicarbonate or baking soda to alter the pH of the terrain of flu patients. And as fate would have it, it turned out to be one of their most effective treatments. Sodium bicarbonate is a base, meaning the opposite of an acid. As such, when administered, it changed the pH of the terrain between cells, making it inhospitable to the Spanish flu.

Sodium bicarbonate is very safe. Once in the body, it breaks down to water and carbon dioxide. Note: There is one very important caveat to remember—never give baking soda to someone with a full stomach because there will be no room for the release of carbon dioxide and you could potentially rupture someone's stomach.

Here is how they dosed their baking soda: The mixture never changed, only the frequency of administration.
Day 1: One-half teaspoon of baking soda in a glass of cold water every two hours for a total of six doses.
Day 2: Same as above, but only a maximum of four doses.
Day 3: Same dose, however, only upon awakening and going to bed.
Day 4 and after: Only once a day every morning.

Another old treatment for the flu was used by the natives of the Pacific Northwest. These local tribes sailed through the Spanish flu of 1918, which decimated local white settlers. The reason was their use of a native herb in the carrot family called *Lomatium dissectum*, or commonly known as fernleaf biscuitroot.

In recent testing, it has been shown to have strong antiviral and antibacterial effects, including the flu and all the respiratory infections mentioned in this chapter—is even deadly to tuberculosis. It even works as an antifungal and is beneficial in the treatment of *Candida albicans* infections.

Scientists have described it as the strongest native antiviral plant in existence. It worked very effectively against the Spanish flu of 1918, so I am very confident that it will work against any flu virus. Especially if you are using this in combination with other treatments like baking soda and also quercetin and zinc to name a few.

This will alter the terrain, making it difficult for viruses to infect cells—and if they do, the quercetin will act as an ionophore, opening a channel into the cell for antiviral zinc to kill any viruses that gained entry. Those three treatments along with general measures to improve your immunity will be incredibly effective at treating any flu virus.

The pH scale

| 0 | 1 | 2 | 3 | 4 | 5 | 6 | 7 | 8 | 9 | 10 | 11 | 12 | 13 | 14 |

acidic   neutral   alkaline

Now, we have our ace in the hole: nebulized hydrogen peroxide and iodine. As described earlier, this is a very effective method of treating any respiratory tract infections from the sinuses and throat to the lungs. As it turns out, it is very effective in treating a flu infection. Always remember to dilute it in saline so the osmolality is similar to body fluids.

You can do a treatment with hydrogen peroxide, enhanced with a drop of iodine, as often as you like. For the flu, I would suggest starting it with every four hours while awake. You can increase it to every two or even every hour if you need to, but it is unlikely you will need it that much.

If you do need it that often, it is not dangerous since hydrogen peroxide breaks down to water and oxygen. As you remember, hydrogen peroxide is directly virucidal or deadly to viruses. It is what the white cells of the body release to kill infections.

As I described earlier, under the bronchitis and pneumonia section, you can nebulize with magnesium chloride and also with iodine drops, both of which are very effective in treating the flu.

If you want to use the natural herbal treatments described earlier in this chapter, you can begin using *Andrographis paniculata* and *Lomatium dissectum*. You can use them alone or together to provide immune stimulation and antiviral activity. The dosing is described earlier under bronchitis and pneumonia. Alternatively or in addition, you can use medicinal mushrooms like reishi and chaga described earlier. Elderberry is also useful in its various forms—once again, described earlier in this chapter.

Don't forget every mother's secret weapon: chicken soup. When there is an old wives' treatment passed down for generations, it is not because it didn't work but rather due to its effectiveness. Chicken soup has a well-earned reputation as a cure for many illnesses, including the flu. Certainly, part of its effect may be in its delivery, that being by a mother who loves you and is doting on you while you are so sick. Drinking this warm, nourishing broth soothes your entire body, filling you with its healing powers.

There is some scientific evidence backing chicken soup as a treatment. It has been shown to decrease inflammation. It has also been shown to mobilize or speed up the movement of mucus, making it easier to cough it up and helping prevent it from blocking airways. It also makes your nose run, but this might benefit a patient by expelling virus-infected mucus from the body. Chicken soup also helps to soothe a raw, sore throat.

Even chicken soup can be made more potent by the addition of some of the following ingredients:

Fresh garlic will not only give it a wonderful flavor enhancement but also will provide much-needed stimulation for the immune system as well as wonderful sulfa-containing compounds. These sulfa-containing compounds are both anti-inflammatory as well as being strong antioxidants.

Mixed vegetables such as organic greens—like collard greens, kale, swiss chard, spinach—onions, potatoes, turnips, and sweet potatoes will all add a host of beneficial phytochemicals or plant nutrients. A pinch of sea salt will add minerals and flavor as well. When adding these ingredients, do so five minutes before the chicken soup is finished cooking. That way you retain the all-important enzymes and flavor.

You can use over-the-counter medications as well. For head congestion, antihistamines are king, as well as nasal sprays such as Afrin, Nasonex, and Flonase. Steam treatments will also help to break up any impacted mucus. Mucinex will work as an expectorant and a decongestant.

The flu is notorious for causing pain, either from headaches or myalgias (muscle aches). Excedrin works great for headaches, oftentimes enhanced when combined with an antihistamine like Benadryl, Zyrtec, Xyzal, Claritin, Allegra, or Clarinex. The use of ice packs to the back of your neck and forehead will also help most headaches.

Other OTC painkillers such as Motrin, Advil, Aleve, and ibuprofen can all be used individually in combination with Tylenol or acetaminophen. For example, take two Tylenols with any two of the others on that list. That is as effective as an opiate painkiller!

Hydration is super important with the flu since it often causes high fevers and fluid loss from sweating, sputum loss, and frequent urination. The result is a very dehydrated patient. If you are dehydrated, your body cannot function properly, especially your immune system. Make a concerted effort to properly hydrate yourself.

Water is the best for this, but you can also use apple juice, unsweetened iced tea, fresh lemons squeezed in water. Do not use coffee or tea, which are diuretics, thus making you urinate and lose even more fluid. Drink a large glass of water upon waking up and two before every meal or every four to six hours while awake and another at bedtime. You will know when you are adequately hydrated by looking at your tongue. If your tongue looks dry, then you need to drink more until your tongue is consistently wet.

Don't forget getting a good-night's sleep. Rest helps every infection by utilizing your body's full energy to fighting the infection. I tell patients to hydrate themselves well and throw on an old sweatshirt and get under that comforter and get a good eight hours plus of sleep—if you can get twelve hours, then do it.

The last thing to remember is to let your fever burn. Unless you go really high, as in above 102 degrees F or more or are delirious, then you will need to lower your fever. Other than that, treating a fever will undermine your body's own best defense to infection. Let it burn; it will shorten the length and severity of your flu.

As you can see, you have many options to treat the flu. You don't need to do all of the above treatments. A handful will probably suffice to eradicate any infection. But certainly, if you wanted to, you could do all of the above. Either way, you should play it by ear, see how you are doing; and if need be, keep adding in various treatments, none of which have any serious side effects.

CHAPTER SEVEN

COVID-19

COVID-19 has unfortunately been the dominant news story for about the last year. It has changed the way we live, work, and socialize. As of the writing of this book, currently the end of February 2021, it has a death rate similar to the seasonal flu. It appears that lots of people are dying with COVID-19 but not necessarily from it. In fact, according to the CDC (Centers for Disease Control and Prevention), only 6 percent of people infected with COVID-19 actually die of it. The other 94 percent are dying with it. Meaning, they have COVID-19, but that is not what is killing them.

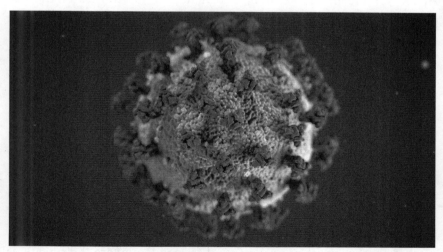

A major part of the problem is the way we are counting COVID-19 deaths here in the United States. If you have a positive COVID-19 test and you die of any other reason, say getting hit by a car, then that is counted as a COVID-19 death! There is a mountain of people who have been falsely diagnosed as being COVID-19 positive. These people do not have COVID-19, but if any of them die, that is now considered a COVID-19 death.

Another huge problem is the test for diagnosing. COVID-19 uses a PCR reaction. It requires amplification of the specimen so it can be interpreted. Kary Mullis was the scientist who won the Nobel Prize in Chemistry for discovering PCR. He said it should never be used as a tool for diagnosis. What it does is amplify very tiny bits of DNA or fragments. Clinically, this is a useless way to determine if someone is infected or not.

Even more insane is the how the current PCR test for COVID-19 was developed. The originators of the PCR test developed the test without a sample of the COVID-19 virus. Since it originated in China, the Chinese hesitated in making available its gene sequences. So, the developers of the PCR test used sequences of other viruses from a gene bank. China finally gave them a genetic sequence with no corresponding viral isolates, hence almost useless.

The other problem with the COVID-19 test is the amplification is too high. It should be less than twenty times, ideally seventeen. Above seventeen, the accuracy and hence the usefulness of the test drops off dramatically. However, it is being used as high as forty-five amplification.

Dr. Mina an epidemiologist at the Harvard T.H. Chan School of Public Health, stated that using an amplification of 45 is "absolutely insane." Because at that mangnification, you may be looking at a single RNA molecule, whereas "When people are sick and contagious, they literally can have one trillion times that number." This is causing up to 80 percent of the tests to be false positives. These are people who do not have COVID-19, have no symptoms, and are not contagious. Yet they are being quarantined under virtual house arrest, are not allowed to work, and are subject to contact tracing. Using these tests, we will have a permanent pandemic!

Yet another problem with this entire "pandemic" are the ridiculous public health recommendations. None of which are grounded in science, even though the powers that be keep stressing that they are following the science.

For example, the social distancing has no scientific study that confirms its usefulness. At the beginning of the outbreak, we were told by Dr. Fauci that we needed to space twenty feet apart. Then they inexplicably lowered that to six feet, once again without any verifiable scientific justification. Dr. Fauci, who doesn't even own a stethoscope and has never practiced medicine, at first scoffed at the need for wearing masks. At least he originally got that right. Then he made an about-face and said we have to wear masks, just for a few weeks until the threat passed.

Now, once again, they have literally doubled down on their earlier recommendation and were now saying we have to wear two masks, and perhaps three would be better. Once again, no science to back it up; and at a certain point, it becomes difficult to breathe through these damn masks.

The reality is masks are almost entirely ineffective. All masks do is protect you from large water droplets, the kind you make when you sneeze. When was the last time someone sneezed right on you and got you wet? Most people answer never. I am a doctor in the trenches seeing patients who are sneezing and coughing every day, and I cannot even remember one time when someone sneezed in my face and got me wet with water droplets.

Dr. Denis Rancourt, a renowned physicist, did a comprehensive review of the world literature on the usefulness of masks to prevent respiratory tract infections such as COVID-19. What he found was astonishing. Studies confirm that surgical masks and even respirators do not prevent transmission of respiratory viruses.

The reason for this is simple: the dominant means of transmission of COVID-19 and other respiratory viruses is from very fine aerosol particles. These aerosol particles are virus particles suspended in air. That is why wearing masks is useless. If the masks allow air to pass through them (which they all do, or you couldn't breathe), then so do the viral particles carrying the disease.

These aerosol particles stay suspended in air when the absolute humidity is low, such as during the winter months. That is why cold, flu, and other respiratory viruses such as corona viruses (such as COVID-19) have a seasonal variability. This is not new information and has been well known for over a decade. For that reason, as you move closer to the equator, the humidity rises, and the transmission of these respiratory illnesses plummet.

Some folks make the argument that the masks are worn to prevent someone infected from spreading his or her infection to healthy people. This too is refuted by the fact that the masks do not stop aerosol particles from going through it, thus they do not confer any form of protection in either direction. Hence they are useless.

Cotton masks and those ridiculous plastic face shields are even more useless than the surgical masks and N95 masks. The pores in the cotton masks are too large to stop any transmission, and the plastic face shields just allow completely unfiltered air to come in from the sides.

Others make the argument that surgeons have worn surgical masks for almost a century in order to protect patients from disease. The reality is that those masks were and are worn to prevent water droplets from falling into the open wound. Nobody ever said they were protecting against viral transmission.

The other mode of viral transmission often mentioned by the breathless, almost-hysterical mainstream news anchors is via fomites. Fomites are objects or material that are likely to carry infection. We have been told that there have been numerous scientific studies showing that viral particles may survive for hours on different types of fomites, such as furniture or doorknobs. However, there has not been even one study confirming that transmission of COVID-19 is possible via fomites.

One very telling detail about this "pandemic" is the lack in rise of "all-cause mortality." All-cause mortality is the total number of people who die in a given year from all causes. This typically would include all types of diseases, suicides, accidents, and in this case, new infections such as the much-touted COVID-19 pandemic.

A war or a new fatal infection would cause a very abrupt spike in the deaths from all-cause mortality. Typically, there is a spike in deaths during the winter months due to all types of respiratory illnesses. During a pandemic such as COVID-19, one would expect a sudden and dramatic spike in deaths. This has not occurred; the death rate is no different than it has been for the last several decades. How can that be if this is such a deadly disease? No one in the government or academia has been able to answer such questions.

The response to COVID-19 in the Western world has been nothing short of insane. For example, it has been proven that children and even young college-age adults rarely get or transmit COVID-19. In the entire United States, the most recent data shows a total of nineteen deaths of school-age children. Nineteen in the entire country! Of those, all nineteen had other serious health conditions such as bad asthma. None of them were healthy.

The year before COVID-19, 180 children died of the flu. Now keep in mind, kids both get the flu and also transmit the flu. So why, pray tell, are we closing schools now, making children wear masks, putting up plexiglass dividers everywhere, and making them space apart? Not to mention spending billions of dollars on new filtration systems for schools. Now they are talking about mass vaccination of school children.

What are we doing? Have we lost our damn minds? We are willing to give an experimental messenger RNA vaccine to our most vulnerable when they don't need it. When we have absolutely no idea of the long-term ramifications of this vaccine.

The incredible harm that closing schools has done to our children is incalculable. Mental health problems among children have skyrocketed. These poor kids are socially isolated and hurting. Suicide is at an all-time high. And why? For a virus that doesn't affect them. Historians will look back in amazement at these incredibly scary times.

Colleges and universities have also, in my opinion, way overreacted to COVID-19. They have cancelled classes and sent students home. They have no activities, sports have been cancelled, no socializing, no working out at the school gym, no concerts, no parties. The problem with this is that college-age students rarely get COVID-19, and if they do get it, their survival rate is 99.992 percent!

Most of the students diagnosed with it are asymptomatic false positives. The students that get it sail through it like a bad cold. What would happen if they left the schools open? Well, we know the answer to that since one sane school decided to stay open. It was Liberty University in Virginia. Appropriately named in my humble opinion. Was there a mass die-off of their student population? Hardly. One student – a commuter – got it and was barely sick at all. They wear masks, but they did not close down, and their students still have a great college experience without the COVID-19 insanity.

Another problem is the so-called vaccine. A *vaccine* by definition is something that confers immunity from a disease, protecting the person from that disease. The current Moderna and Pfizer vaccines do neither. Both companies admit that the vaccine does not protect you from getting COVID-19, it just lessens the severity of your symptoms! By the way, it also does not prevent you from transmitting the disease. You still shed viral particles and are contagious.

According to a former vice president and chief scientific adviser for one of the vaccine manufacturers, Pfizer, named Dr. Michael Yeadon, very few people will need the COVID-19 vaccine as the mortality rate so low and the illness is clearly not causing excessive deaths. He also noted the lack of a spike in all-cause mortality and said, "You cannot have a lethal pandemic stalking the land and not have excess deaths."

So, what good is it? The bad news is that they are selling this as a "vaccine" when in fact, it is actually gene therapy. Gene therapy would be a very hard sell to the public, but vaccines, they are accustomed to. What do I mean by gene therapy? The COVID-19 "vaccines" use a novel method—they use messenger RNA or mRNA.

The theory is that injecting messenger RNA will direct the cell's DNA to change and start producing the SARS-CoV-2 spike protein. Your immune system will detect the presence of this viral protein and will begin producing antibodies. The problem is that this is a theory, and unfortunately, it has not undergone the usual animal testing.

Therefore we have no way of knowing both the short-term and long-term side effects of this novel vaccine. In the past, when they tried other coronavirus vaccines, the animals initially did well with a robust immune response. However, later when infected with the same coronavirus or other respiratory pathogens, all the animals died via a process known as antibody dependent enhancement (ADE). ADE is a damaging inflammatory reaction triggered by their own antibodies binding to their own cells and tissues and depositing immune complexes. This inflammatory cascade ultimately proved to be universally fatal to those lab animals.

Another huge concern is the mass vaccination of women of childbearing age. The "vaccine" directs the cells of your body to produce this spike protein on their surfaces. The problem is that similar spike proteins are essential in the formation of the human placenta. If the body is attacking these proteins, there is a good chance that it will also interfere with the formation of a placenta. This has the potential to induce mass infertility in an entire generation of Western women getting this vaccine.

These new vaccines from Pfizer and Moderna contain lipid nanoparticles that contain polyethylene glycol to deliver the mRNA into the cell. This delivery system has never been approved for use in any vaccine or drug.

Originally, in 2017, Moderna tried to use lipid nanoparticles in an effort to treat a rare disease. They abandoned using this technology due to adverse reactions from the patient's immune systems. These lipid nanoparticles also cross the blood-brain barrier and freely enter the brain. The blood-brain barrier is a filtering mechanism of the capillaries that carry blood to the brain and spinal cord. It is meant to prevent foreign and harmful substances from entering the brain. No one knows the long-term side effects of lipid nanoparticles on the central nervous system (brain and spinal cord).

If all that was not bad enough, manufacturers of the vaccine have been granted total immunity from any liability caused by their vaccines.

The real crime is that for all but a few cohorts of patients, vaccines for COVID-19 are not needed. When one takes into consideration its overall low lethality and weigh that against an experimental vaccine that has not had animal testing and its potential harm and even lethality, it fails to justify the vaccine for all but a few groups of very elderly or very sick patients.

It is becoming increasingly clear that maintaining certain nutrients will confer better protection than a vaccine. Those nutrients are the ones I have been talking about in this entire book. They are what I like to call the gang of seven, which includes vitamins A, C, and D; zinc; iodine; selenium; and quercetin. Why expose yourself to the risk of gene therapy, permanently changing every cell in your body with its unknown long-term consequences, when you can protect yourself with nutrients that have nothing but beneficial side effects?

Even more disturbing is the total ostracization of anyone who questions the narrative that we have been fed about COVID-19. If they are physicians, they are tossed out of academic institutions, their licenses are revoked, and they are called conspiracy theorists. Even renowned physicians such as Dr. Joseph Mercola, who for many years has had the most popular alternative medical website on the Internet, has been demonetized and marginalized by the powers that be.

Why, you ask? Because he has been honest and courageous enough to do exactly what a good physician or scientist should do, that is question any theory and provide evidence for the dissenting opinion. In present-day America and the entire Western world, that has become a reason to destroy your livelihood and completely trash your reputation. Why are they so afraid of any discussion or debate over this virus?

My humble opinion is that this virus is being used as an excuse for governments to exert greater political control and to usher in what is known as the Great Reset. It is beyond the scope of this book, but look it up, it will blow your mind. I would refer you to Armstrong Economics at armstrongeconomics.com for an excellent analysis of the Great Reset and its ominous goals as it plays out in real time.

By the way, I am not saying that COVID-19 is not real or not deadly for many people. The seasonal flu is deadly for a lot of people. What I am saying is that it is not the killer that it is made out to be. I believe the reaction to it is not only unwarranted but oftentimes totally ineffective and not ground in good science or medicine.

Okay, that is enough of my rant on COVID-19. Let's now take a look at how to prevent it and how to treat it if you do come down with it.

PREVENTION OF COVID-19

Handwashing is still and always will be an excellent tool in the prevention of all respiratory tract diseases. People tend to cough into their hands and then grab a doorknob or touch other areas. Uninfected people either shake hands with the infected person or touch a doorknob or other surface and get the virus on their hands. We constantly touch our faces with our hands and thus transmit the virus to our nose and mouth, where it gains entry into our bodies. That is why health-care workers are always washing their hands between patients: in order to protect themselves and others from disease transmission.

Personal hygiene is crucial to good health and should not be overlooked. Cleaning your body and brushing your teeth regularly helps eliminate a large burden of pathogens trying to get a foothold on your body. One iron-clad rule I can state with confidence is that I have never seen a patient with really bad teeth in good health. The two just don't go together. Rotten teeth and infected gums seed their bodies with an endless stream of pathogens and the toxins they produce. Eventually, their bodies succumb to this endless onslaught, and chronic diseases are the result.

Another effective way to prevent all respiratory tract infections including COVID-19 is to use a mouthwash. The common dental mouthwashes sold in stores will work just fine for this purpose. Brands such as ACT, Listerine, Crest mouthwash, TheraBreath, and Colgate Peroxyl all will work for our purposes. The active ingredients that we are looking for include ethanol, chlorhexidine, hydrogen peroxide, and povidone-iodine, to name a few.

How these mouthwashes work is by inactivation of COVID-19 by destroying the fat or lipid layer that surrounds the virus, thus preventing it from reproducing itself.

You can also sterilize your toothbrushes by using a combination of Listerine and the 3 percent hydrogen peroxide commonly found in pharmacies and grocery stores. Fill a small glass with this mix and immerse your toothbrushes in it and swish it around. Leave them in there for a few minutes and they will be sterilized.

Alternative methods of disinfecting your toothbrush are to soak it in any of the above mouthwashes alone for thirty seconds, dissolve two teaspoons of baking soda in a cup of water and soak the toothbrush in this for five minutes, or dissolve a denture-cleaning tablet in a glass of water and soak the toothbrush in it for several minutes.

You can also fill a small glass with water and put four drops of iodine such as Betadine, Lugol's solution, or nascent iodine, and let the toothbrush soak in that for a few minutes. Any of the above methods will work, but I personally think the iodine solution is the most potent of all.

IVERMECTIN

One very effective albeit controversial method of both preventing and treating COVID-19 is ivermectin. Ivermectin is a very well-known, FDA-approved treatment for parasitic infections such as onchocerciasis or river blindness. Incredibly, it was found in the soil adjacent to a golf course in Japan in 1975 by a Japanese scientist and has never been found again anywhere on Earth! Talk about a gift from God.

It has been used since the 1970s and has a long track record of both safety and efficacy. There have been reports of its usefulness against many viral infections, and due to this, once again, the inquisitive doctors of the medical underground have resurrected it in their fight against COVID-19. One such group is the Front Line COVID-19 Critical Care Alliance or FLCCC. Don't ask me why it is not called the FLCCCA? That doesn't bother me as much as the fact that we call people with orange hair redheads; however, once again, I digress.

They have a wonderful website which is a gold mine of medical information on the prevention and treatment of COVID-19, and I encourage all my readers to go there and review their wonderful articles and research papers.

The FLCCC was organized in response to the COVID-19 pandemic in March 2020. They are a world-renowned collection of highly published medical researchers and clinicians supported by physicians "in the trenches" all over the world. They have developed treatment protocols that have saved tens of thousands of patients worldwide and have now set their sights on prevention.

They have identified ivermectin as the key medication for the prevention of COVID-19. Ivermectin is a very safe medication and has been recognized by the WHO as one of mankind's essential medications and has been administered over 3.7 billion times!

Ivermectin works by inhibiting the replication of COVID-19, flu, and apparently many other viruses. It also acts to quell the inflammation caused by pieces COVID-19 viral RNA, lowers viral loads (the amount of virus in the blood), protects against organ damage, and most importantly, it lowers the risk of hospitalization and death. Ivermectin also has been demonstrated to prevent transmission of COVID-19 when taken before or even after exposure!

Inflammation has been identified as one of the primary causes of morbidity (sickness) and mortality from COVID-19. The doctors of the FLCCC are using ivermectin in all stages of COVID-19. It is as of yet unapproved by the NIH; however, the wheels of power move slowly, and in January 2021, they changed their stance from "against" to "neutral."

We, docs of the medical underground, moved ahead on our own since patients were dying and mainstream medicine had nothing to offer, and even more strangely, politics was coming into play in a major way, suppressing any medical opinions that weren't the official "party line." That was a very terrifying first for many of us since in our training, we were encouraged to debate with those of differing medical opinions in an open forum, where the best ideas rose to the top.

That, sadly, is no longer the case in the United States, where we used to be the land of the free and the home of the brave, but now are the land of the censored and the home of the coerced.

Here are their recommendations for the prevention of COVID-19:

Ivermectin: For high-risk patients, 0.2 mg/per kilogram of body weight (1 kg = 2.2 lbs) one dose day one, repeat in two days, and again one week later. For non-high-risk patients, same 0.2 mg/kg, but one dose now and a second after two days. Note: for most patients, this works out roughly to 6 mg to 12 mg of ivermectin. It is usually manufactured in 3 mg, 6 mg, and 12 mg doses.

Vitamin D3: 1,000 to 3,000 international units/daily.

Vitamin C: 500 to 1,000 mg twice daily.

Quercetin: 250 mg/day.

Zinc: 30-40 mg/day.

Melatonin: 6 mg at bedtime (since it makes you tired). Melatonin has anti-inflammatory, antioxidant and immunomodulating effects that help prevent and treat COVID-19. It has proven quite helpful in reducing mortality in hospitalized intubated COVID-19 patients in the ICU. A very interesting fact is that bats have incredibly high levels of melatonin in their blood, possibly as protection from coronaviruses since they are its natural reservoir in the wild. As I mentioned earlier, what I like to call the gang of seven are the most potent for this purpose and include vitamins A, C, and D; zinc; iodine; selenium; and quercetin. However, as I taught you earlier, they are your foundation from which you can layer on other treatments as you need them.

Now, let's take a look at the optimal way to prevent COVID-19 in those of us who do not have access to prescription medications such as ivermectin.

As with all disease, the best way to shield yourself is to supercharge your immune system using the immune-boosting nutrients that I outlined in chapter 5. From the medical underground, a handful of nutrients have emerged that are specifically useful in the prevention of COVID-19. As I mentioned earlier, the ones I think are most potent for this purpose include vitamins A, C, and D3, along with quercetin, zinc, iodine, and selenium. However, as I taught you in chapter 5, these are just the tip of the iceberg.

Only if you think you have been exposed to COVID-19 but are still negative then do the following: If you are not already on any nutraceuticals to boost your immunity, then jump-start it with the seven I mentioned above. Start off with small doses for now. If you convert to positive, then we will ramp up all of them. For now, start with the following:

Vitamin C. Start with 1 gram (1,000 mg) twice a day. Remember, it is water soluble and can be taken on an empty stomach or with food. If you are using the liposomal version of vitamin C, that is fat soluble and best to be taken with a fatty meal. The dose on that is usually around 1,200 mg daily. Once a day should suffice. Vitamin C is a potent antiviral; it works against all viruses; you just have to give enough of it.

The good news is that is completely nontoxic and safe. Nobody has ever died from a vitamin C overdose.

Vitamin D3. You should start with a minimum of 5,000 international units (IUs) or 7,500 IUs daily. It is very important to remember to take this with a fatty meal to ensure its proper absorption. Many recent studies confirm the usefulness of vitamin D3 in both the prevention and the treatment of COVID-19. Remember, exposing yourself to adequate sunlight without any sunblock for short periods every day will go a long way to raising your vitamin D levels. The lower your vitamin D levels in your blood, the greater your risk of contracting respiratory tract infections, especially flu and COVID-19. Remember that vitamin D is more like a hormone than a vitamin, with extensive collateral benefits for your entire body.

Vitamin A. Vitamin A is another fat-soluble vitamin, just like vitamins D and E. Vitamin A helps support the proper function of both the innate and adaptive immune systems as well as many of our organs such as the heart, kidneys, and lungs. Vitamin A helps increase the production of antibodies by the immune system and also increases interferon and natural killer immune cells. If you want your respiratory tract to function optimally, you need adequate vitamin A.

Inflammation and infections are both treated by vitamin A, especially respiratory tract infections such as the flu and COVID-19. Vitamin A is found in multiple food sources such as dairy products, fish, meat, and especially in liver. Liver is where vitamin A is stored in most animals. Liver is the food with the highest vitamin A content, therefore eating liver is a wonderful way to get your vitamin A.

Cod liver oil is my second favorite way of getting your vitamin A. I love the taste of fish, so for me, it is no problem. However, for those of you that don't, no worries, they now have lemon-flavored cod-liver oil. It actually tastes quite good, without much of a fishy taste. Remember to keep your cod liver oil refrigerated between uses.

For my vegetarian readers, other good sources of vitamin A are sweet potatoes, pumpkins, spinach, and carrots. Since vitamin A is fat soluble like vitamin D, you need to avoid excessive intake to avoid toxicity. For an acute COVID-19 infection exposure, take 100,000 units of vitamin A daily for five days. After, to avoid toxicity you show, then lower it to once a week, always with a fatty meal to ensure its absorption.

Zinc. If you think you have been exposed or if you feel that you may be "coming down with something," then start taking zinc immediately. Zinc is effective against all viral infections. I would start with 50 mg of chelated zinc daily with food. Food will help increase your absorption of zinc or any other mineral. If you have zinc lozenges (they usually come in around 20 mg doses), suck on two or three a day on a full stomach. If you are starting zinc, it is best to take it along with quercetin.

Quercetin. Quercetin is a flavonoid pigment found in many plants. In many studies, it has been shown to be a potent antiviral, antioxidant, anti-inflammatory, and immune-system booster. Vitamin C helps to regenerate quercetin, thus they work synergistically (mutually helping one another).

Quercetin, vitamin C, vitamin D3, and zinc work as a team as potent antivirals and, as such, should all be taken together at the first sign of an illness. Their activity is not exclusively against COVID-19; they work against all viruses. I will describe this in greater detail later on in this chapter.

Iodine. Iodine comes in many forms. Kelp is the most natural form of iodine and is recognized by your body as a food. Kelp is a giant brown seaweed that grows in "forests" along the coasts. In addition to iodine, it contains antioxidant vitamins A, C, and E.

As a food, it is easily assimilated by your body. That being said, all forms of iodine are well absorbed—you can even apply it to your skin, and it will be absorbed. For our purposes, start with a capsule that provides you with at least 250 mcg of iodine (25 mg).

In my experience, most patients have very low iodine levels, secondary to eating foods grown on depleted soils. For that reason, I would take 25 mg a day to help raise your body's iodine levels. I would not go on higher doses, thinking more is better, because higher doses may suppress thyroid function.

If you are using nascent iodine, then add ten drops a day in a glass of water. Swish it around your mouth and between your teeth and then swallow it. This way, you get the dual effect of disinfecting your mouth and also raising your body's iodine level.

Other forms of iodine are Lugol's solution, mix six drops of this in a glass of water and also swish it around your mouth and then swallow it. Some will be absorbed directly through the mucosa or lining of your mouth into your blood. Another form of iodine is Iodoral. These tablets usually come in 12.5 mg strength. One a day usually suffices to meet your iodine needs and to protect you from ionizing radiation damage to your thyroid. For our purposes, 12.5 mg should suffice. Iodine is deadly to all types of microbes and will greatly assist your immune system.

Selenium. Selenium is a trace mineral that has antioxidant activity as well as acting as an immune system booster. Selenium is also a component of many enzymes and is essential to proper thyroid function. One of the most important of those selenium-dependent enzymes is glutathione reductase, which is responsible for tissue repair.

In other words, it helps your body heal itself, especially after an infection. Start off with selenium 200 mcg once a day with food to help increase its absorption. This will provide your body with a readily available pool of selenium in order to defend itself.

THE GANG OF SEVEN

Note: Always remember to reach for the gang of seven—iodine, zinc, quercetin, selenium, vitamin A, vitamin C, and vitamin D3—whenever you suspect you have a viral infection of any type. The gang of seven works against *all viruses.* Just to be clear, the gang of seven will help boost your immune system and will help with *any infection,* but they are especially effective against viral infections where there are not many other treatment options currently available.

The gang of seven, in combination, will block viral entry into the cell, viral protein formation, and most importantly viral replication. There are no prescription drugs that can do that. The added bonus is that they have nothing but beneficial side effects. These nutrients have been used by the medical underground for years and have proven to be quite effective and exceedingly safe.

The pharmaceutical companies would be putting everyone in the world on them if they could patent them! They have nothing that compares to the efficacy and safety of the gang of seven!

Now, those nutrients are a wonderful start in helping your immune system meet the challenge of either an exposure to COVID-19 or a full-blown infection that is in its early stages. As with any sickness, the first few days are critical to help your body. I cannot overemphasize the importance of a good long (at least eight hours) night of deep, uninterrupted sleep, along with good hydration.

Drink two glasses of water when you wake up and two before every meal and one or two at bedtime. Use your tongue as a barometer of your hydration. Look in the mirror—if your tongue is wet, you are well hydrated; if not, continue to drink water. Sleep, hydration, and the gang of seven, will go a long way to strengthening your body for the fight ahead.

YOUR MENTAL ATTITUDE

One thing that I have not mentioned so far is your mental attitude. If there is one thing I have learned in my many decades in practice, it is that attitude is everything. When I have had the unfortunate task of informing a patient that they have cancer, they immediately split into two groups. One group immediately becomes determined to beat the cancer and are aggressive and optimistic that it will not "get them." I have learned from experience that this group will do much better, no matter what stage of cancer they are diagnosed with.

The second group almost collapses upon the news of a cancer diagnosis. They immediately begin to feel sorry for themselves and become deeply depressed and pessimistic. They roll over and, for the most part, accept the fact that they are "screwed" and are going to die, and they do. They die faster and more horribly than their upbeat counterparts. They suffer through each stage of their decline until they succumb. They undermine their own immune system with their negativity and, in effect, doom themselves.

The public has no conception as to the extent of the mind's control over our bodies. That is why I say that attitude is everything. If you are depressed, guess what, so is your immune system. If you are upbeat and laughing at life, your immune system will follow. We are not separate from our immune system—it is us. It is our very essence. That is why our moods have such a direct effect. Medical studies for decades have confirmed the mind-body connection. People who are going through a life crisis, such as death of a child, parent, or spouse, have much higher rates of illness, with much worse outcomes.

A great example of my "attitude is everything" belief comes from Norman Cousins's wonderful book, *Anatomy of an Illness*. Mr. Cousins was the editor of the *Saturday Review*. In the mid-1960s, he came down with an incredibly painful case of ankylosing spondylitis. He was bedridden and racked with pain. After much suffering, he decided to end all painkillers and check himself out of the hospital and into a hotel room with a nurse.

Haven't we all had that fantasy? However, once again, I digress. He went on high-dose vitamin C, and she read funny stories to him, and they watched old comedy films and television series. He found that ten minutes of solid laughter gave him about two hours of drug-free pain relief. Eventually, he became free of painkillers and sleeping pills and went on to be completely cured.

That form of treatment has now been recognized by the American Medical Association as laughter therapy. His book is inspiring and a great read. I love this quote of his:

"The greatest force in the human body is the natural drive for the body to heal itself. But that force is not independent of the belief system. What we believe is the most powerful option of all. The control center of your life is your attitude."

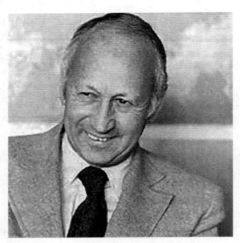

Norman Cousins

For myself, a large part of my attitude comes from my belief in God. I have a belief system that encompasses a wonderful, loving God that not only wants to help you but is willing to sacrifice his only son for you! When you believe in God, he is all in for you. Once you have a grounding in a strong belief in God, you are never alone in your fight. In fact, you have the Creator of the entire universe on your side. How much better can it get than that?

Hopefully, I have convinced you that a spiritual, upbeat, positive attitude filled with laughter and optimism will go a very long way to keeping you healthy and happy. There is absolutely no downside to it. What have you got to lose? Nothing will serve your needs better than the belief that you will remain healthy, and if you do happen to get sick that you will recover rapidly without any ill aftereffects.

SYMPTOMS OF COVID-19

According to the CDC, the most common symptoms are fever, dry cough, and fatigue. The vast majority of the patients that I have treated with COVID-19 really emphasize the fatigue. They are wiped out, falling asleep at their desks at work before their official diagnosis, falling asleep while driving, sleeping for twelve to sixteen hours straight without waking. I am talking about absolute exhaustion.

This state of extreme fatigue is followed almost immediately by the beginning of a dry cough. I have found that the patients who are not going to do well and will need hospitalization rapidly develop dyspnea or shortness of breath. It is rapid and scary for them, and they wind up in the hospital shortly thereafter.

Fever accompanies their other symptoms at this stage, and here is where most people make a serious mistake: they treat the fever. They immediately begin taking aspirin or Tylenol because they are foolishly worried about a fever, unaware that it is their body's greatest defense against an infection.

One of the greatest hallmarks of a COVID-19 infection is the loss of taste and smell. There are very few infections that cause a loss of taste and smell; for this reason, quite correctly, the public associates it with COVID-19.

Diseases of the sinuses and nose can cause a loss of smell, but not usually taste. Head colds frequently stuff up the nose and prevent olfaction (your sense of smell). Head trauma can also cause loss of olfaction but, once again, does not usually involve taste. If you have lost both, you very likely have COVID-19.

Pain is another symptom, usually generalized muscle aches or a headache. In my experience, the headache is not severe. Either one usually will respond to over-the-counter pain relievers such as Excedrin, Aleve, Motrin, Advil, and ibuprofen.

Other common symptoms are a sore, scratchy throat, dizziness, runny nose, diarrhea, nausea, vomiting and possibly a red skin rash. Sometimes there is a red discoloration of the toes, now known as COVID toes. Sometimes, the toes are painful as well. Inflammation of your eyes, causing them to be sensitive and reddened, is also a manifestation, usually with no loss of visual acuity (eyesight).

The CDC reports the following symptoms as serious enough to require immediate emergency medical evaluation: trouble breathing, persistent chest pain or pressure in the chest, confusion, the inability to stay awake or be awoken, and pale gray or bluish discoloration of lips, skin and/or nail beds depending upon skin tone. All these symptoms are indicative of respiratory failure, with resulting low oxygen levels and or cardiac or neurological involvement. All of which are medical emergencies and have to be immediately evaluated by a physician.

TREATMENT OF COVID-19

Let's now take a look at the worst-case scenario and you have caught COVID-19. First of all, unless you are in your eighties and/or have a list of comorbidities, this is probably going to be nothing worse than a run-of-the-mill cold or flu. There is a very good chance that you will sail through it with very little or no symptoms. That being said, it does randomly take out adults who otherwise appear to be in good health of all ages. So, in no way should it be minimalized as a disease; however, statistics do paint a much rosier picture where in almost every demographic, except the very old or those with multiple comorbidities, the survival rate of those infected with COVID-19 is north of 99 percent! As doctors gain more experience treating it, those numbers continue to improve.

Note: None of the treatments that I am describing are cures for COVID-19. These treatments will all help alleviate your symptoms and hopefully hasten your recovery. Like all viral respiratory tract infections, there are no official known cures for any of them, and the FDA seriously comes down on any doctor that says there are. That being said, let's look at some great ways to treat a COVID-19 infection that have arisen from the medical underground!

START WITH THE GANG OF SEVEN

If you skipped the first part of this chapter, first of all, shame on you, but that being said, you should go back and immediately begin doing all the things I recommended earlier. Immediately, get a lot of rest and hydration. Start the gang of seven essential immune boosters that I recommended. Take them for five days and then go to the full doses of those vitamins and minerals. The only exceptions are dosing of vitamins A, C, and D3.

Vitamin A will help balance your immune response and decrease deadly inflammation and the cytokine storm that accompanies

COVID-19. Keeping in mind that like vitamin D, it is fat-soluble, hence we have to be careful of toxicity with long-term high-dose administration. For that reason, I want you to take 100,000 international units daily for the first five days then lower it to once a week thereafter. That should adequately boost your vitamin A stores and provide enough for proper function of your immune system and your respiratory tract.

Vitamin D3 is proving to be one of the most important natural treatments for both prevention and treatment of COVID-19. For that reason, I would recommend immediately starting very high doses of it for the first five days or so. I am talking about doses in the 50,000 international units daily with fat for the first five days.

After that, take the same dose twice a week until you are better. When you are cured, reduce it to once a week—remember, always with a fatty meal so you absorb it. In a recent study, 98.9 percent of patients with vitamin D levels below 20 ng/ml died from COVID-19! Mainstream doctors use 30 ng/ml as a normal vitamin D level, which is totally wrong. The ideal level is between 60-80 ng/ml. It is without side effects up to a blood level of 100 ng/ml. If the weather is good, get out in the sun; this will naturally raise your vitamin D level as well as make you feel much better.

Vitamin C is the other vitamin that is absolutely critical to beating COVID-19. Vitamin C is the ultimate virus killer. When adequately dosed, it has been shown to be effective against all types of viruses, with no exceptions. If you are not on it, you should start immediately with 2,000 mg twice a day, double this dose every two days.

Vitamin C is completely harmless. There is no known toxicity. In fact, it is safer than water! The only side effect it has is at high doses, it may cause some diarrhea. If that happens, go back to the previous dose. If it persists, lower it again to the prior dose. That is known as bowel tolerance.

The diarrhea problem can be avoided by using liposomal vitamin C, which is fat soluble. It is very well absorbed and does not cause bowel problems. Its absorption is so high that it is almost comparable to intravenous vitamin C, which is the goal standard for treatment but is not available to the average person.

Here is where you either are going to pat yourself on the back or kick yourself in the butt. Did you buy the nebulizer machine and the supplies you needed to go with it, like the hydrogen peroxide, iodine, and masks for adults and if need be, for your children? Hopefully, by this time in an outbreak, the stores have not been stripped of what you need.

NEBULIZATION

I want you to start your nebulizer treatments ASAP. Nothing will do more to treat COVID-19 or any other respiratory tract infection. Hopefully, you will have the iodine to add to your mix of hydrogen peroxide and saline. Give yourself a treatment every four hours while you are awake.

There is no need to get up during the night unless you are having bouts of coughing and cannot sleep. Adjust the schedule of your treatments to your needs. Remember, as described earlier in the previous chapter in the section on bronchitis and pneumonia, you can also nebulize with magnesium chloride and with iodine diluted in saline.

All these treatments will work against COVID-19 and virtually every respiratory tract infection. Remember, you do not necessarily have to dilute your 3 percent hydrogen peroxide, you can use it at full strength. That is where it will be most potent at killing any infecting microorganisms. If you have any burning sensation in your nose, sinuses, and throat, then I would dilute it. Dilution should always be done with normal saline (salt water) since this is most similar to other body fluids.

Now is a good time to introduce zinc into the treatment regimen. Zinc is very efficient at killing viruses. the drawback is that it must gain access to the inside of the cell or cytoplasm in order to eradicate viral infections. The reason for this is the virus needs to enter the cell so it can take over the DNA in the cell nucleus to make copies of itself. Once enough copies are made, it will stretch the cell enough to explode it, thus expelling all these new virus particles, which now go on to infect healthy cells.

Hydroxychloroquine is the generic name for the drug that goes by the trade name Plaquenil. It became infamous during the height of the pandemic when President Trump rightly touted it as a good treatment for COVID-19. Of course, the mainstream media immediately hated it, thus maintaining their "Orange Man Bad" policy. However, it is a very safe medication that I and thousands of other physicians used for rheumatoid arthritis and lupus for decades without any harmful side effects.

At first, doctors were using it without zinc, then they realized its effectiveness was definitely tied to giving it with zinc. The reason is simple, Plaquenil is an ionophore, meaning it opens an ion channel in the cell membrane, allowing zinc to pass into the cell's interior or cytoplasm. The cell membrane has a positive charge as does zinc, hence it repels zinc. Remember from grade school science, like charges repel and opposites attract.

Viruses have to enter cells in order to take control of the cell's DNA, which is inside the cell's nucleus. In order to fight these infections, you need to get inside the cell. Plaquenil allows the zinc to enter the cell by forming a channel or passageway though the cell membrane into the cytoplasm.

Plaquenil is a prescription medication. Fortunately for our needs, we have another ionophore that is not a prescription medication, called quercetin. Quercetin does the exact same thing as Plaquenil—it opens up the cell for zinc to enter and kill the virus. Therefore you should start taking quercetin 500 mg to 1,000 mg daily and 50 mg of zinc for each 500 mg of quercetin.

There are now quercetin and zinc capsules available that makes it even easier. Make sure your combination pill has 50 mg of zinc and at least 500 mg of quercetin—that will provide enough killing power. There are even some combination pills that contain vitamin D3, vitamin C, quercetin, and zinc! You got to love capitalism—markets are so efficient, they fill every demand, no other economic system can compare.

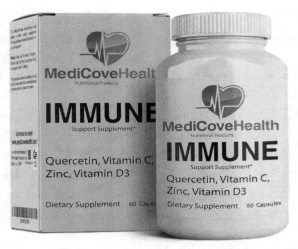

There appears to be almost no side effects from taking quercetin long term at high doses. Studies of patients taking 1 gram (1,000 mg) of quercetin daily for three months reported very few cases of temporary tingling of their legs and mild headaches.

WHY THE GANG OF SEVEN WORK AGAINST ALL VIRAL INFECTIONS

Viruses have to do several things in order to infect us. They must attach to their target cell. Then they must penetrate the wall and get into the cell interior or cytoplasm. After which, they must penetrate the nucleus in order to take over the cell's DNA.

Once inside the DNA, the virus directs it to make copies of its genetic material or genome and also the structural proteins that coat the genome in a shell known as the viral capsid. The genome and the viral capsid proteins self-assemble into new viral particles or virions until there are so many of them the cell explodes, spreading the virus to adjacent cells and so on and so on.

Wouldn't it be incredible to have "medicine" that would block the action of viruses at every one of those stages, as well as balancing your immune response? Well, I have something better for you. How about a team of vitamin, mineral, and plant products that is completely safe and in fact has many wonderful collateral benefits with virtually no side effects? The gang of seven: vitamins A, C, and D3, iodine, quercetin, selenium, and zinc do just that and much more.

That is why the gang of seven should be the first things you should reach for whenever you are starting to get sick. There is absolutely no downside and lots of upside. The odds of developing a serious viral infection plummet when you block the virus at every stage of its development. You are giving yourself nebulizer treatments as frequently as you need, and you are supplementing with iodine, quercetin, selenium, and zinc.

The key to using them is to start treatment as soon as possible. Early treatment blocks viral replication, and thus its spread. Starting this regimen late in an infection severely limits its usefulness.

Now at this point, you are hopefully well hydrated and well rested. You have vastly increased your vitamins, minerals to stimulate as well as properly balance your immune system. You have titrated up your doses of vitamins A, C, and D. You are giving yourself nebulizer treatments as frequently as you need, and you are on iodine, quercetin, and zinc.

Your next step is to begin treating specific symptoms. If you have fever, ignore it unless you are delirious or it is above 102.5 degrees F. In those cases, you can treat it, but for the shortest time possible. You don't want to undermine one of your body's greatest defense mechanisms to infection by stopping your fever.

There is no known treatment for loss of smell and taste; however, I would think that nebulizer treatments would help directly eradicate infections in the affected areas and might very well hasten your recovery.

Fatigue will eventually resolve, but it takes time. Your body is exhausted from fighting off this invasive viral infection. As I have said many times, resting every day during this infection will go a long way to curing it. Also, hydrating yourself is critically important at every stage of this illness. According to Harvard Medical School, when your body is low on fluids, it causes you to feel tired and weaker than normal.

Besides drinking water and other fluids, include eating fruit and vegetables that contain vast amounts of water, which is actually very different from normal water in its makeup, construction, and function in the body and is known as structured water. Soups can also be very nourishing and hydrating, and now is a great time to have some chicken soup, just as you are starting to feel like a truck hit you!

Now is the time to rest. Put on your favorite pajama pants and that old, stained sweatshirt your wife always wants to throw out. Curl up with a good book or watch an old movie, preferably a comedy to get in some laugh therapy, and enjoy that hot bowl of delicious chicken soup.

Pain is not a major symptom of COVID-19. There are headaches and myalgias or muscle aches associated with COVID-19 infections, but they are not a major hallmark of the illness. That is good because any of the pain medications that we would use all reduce fever. I would much rather let your fever burn than inadvertently treating it because you had pain and wanted to take a pain reliever.

All the over-the-counter painkillers are antipyretics or fever reducers. If your muscle pain is bad, use ice packs on it. You can also use Voltaren gel. Voltaren or diclofenac is a nonsteroidal like the other painkillers mentioned above (with the exception of Tylenol) and can potentially reduce fevers, but you are using it topically, and hence it is unlikely to have a systemic effect like reducing your fever.

Voltaren gel should be rubbed on briskly to the painful area for about fifteen seconds up to four times a day. The heat from your hand will help its penetration and absorption.

Voltaren gel works very well for those aches and pains you get with COVID-19 and other viral infections. Other topical pain gels you can use are IcyHot cream, Biofreeze pain relief gel and Salonpas deep-relieving gel, all of which will work just fine.

Headaches can also be treated with ice packs. I find it works best to use two ice packs, one on the back of your neck and the other on your forehead. If you don't have ice packs available, a bag of frozen food from your freezer will suffice. I would advise wrapping it in a paper towel to prevent damaging your skin.

If you have severe pain or headaches, you can also use a combination of two Tylenol with two of either Advil, ibuprofen, or Motrin. That combination is as strong as an opioid analgesic (painkiller). Excedrin also is a very effective headache remedy. Excedrin is made of aspirin, caffeine, and Tylenol. Once again, keep in mind that you should use any of the above pain meds as sparingly as possible if you have a fever.

Head congestion and/or a runny nose can be treated using steam treatments as described previously, with either a steam machine or making a tent with a large towel and putting your head over a sink with hot steamy water running or over a boiling pot of water. Be very careful not to burn yourself. Antihistamines such as Allegra, Benadryl, Claritin, Clarinex, Zyrtec, and Xyzal will all work to decongest you.

Nasal sprays such as Flonase, Nasonex, saline sprays, and Afrin will all work very well to open up a clogged nose. Remember, you can only use Afrin for a week before it causes rebound. Rebound means the congestion will return faster and faster, and eventually, the medication will not work very well. For a week, it is the best at opening up your nose and sinuses.

The Mucinex family of products won't work very well to clear up your head congestion; however, they work wonderfully to break up chest congestion.

Nebulizer treatments will also help head congestion and a runny nose by treating the virus directly and will also help to break up chest congestion.

Nausea and vomiting are more difficult symptoms to treat. If you have an antiemetic (nausea and vomiting medication) such as Zofran (ondansetron) or Compazine (prochlorperazine), now is the time to use them. Marijuana works wonderfully for the relief of nausea and vomiting and has been used to treat cancer patients undergoing chemotherapy for decades.

You can smoke it or use edibles—either one will work. CBD oil will also work to help nausea and vomiting. So, get out your bong or roll a couple of doobies and toke up. However, having said that, I would smoke as little as possible since any smoke, whether tobacco or marijuana, will irritate your lungs and may increase your coughing.

We are all adults; determine what is more important for you: alleviating nausea and vomiting or your cough. And choose your treatment accordingly. I am here to guide you through your sickness and give you an entire host of treatment options for you to choose from.

Forget about nonsense like getting into a full lotus position, putting a pyramid-shaped hat on your head, and chanting of mantras with incense burning. I have been a practicing physician for over three decades, I am not preaching to you from an ivory tower.

I have been in the trenches treating patients in emergency rooms, hospitals, prisons, clinics, nursing homes, at the VA, and in my private practice. I have made it my life's work to find the most effective traditional and alternative treatments from the medical underground. There are many old remedies that work quite well; things like Epsom salts, honey, and baking soda can go a long way toward healing many afflictions. Let's take a look at one of my favorites.

BAKING SODA

Baking soda, as I taught you in the previous chapter, was used very successfully to treat the Spanish flu of 1918. Changing the extracellular spaces pH has a profound effect against most respiratory viruses since most require an acidic pH to bind to their target cells. The necessity of an acidic pH is a target we can exploit. Here is an opportunity to literally block the enemy at the gates.

If the virus cannot penetrate the cell membrane, it cannot survive and reproduce. What a brilliant strategy. If you do this along with the gang of seven, it will give you a superweapon against viruses by blocking the viral attachment to the cell membrane. Then if any viral particles get through into the cell, you have all the virucidal (virus killing) effects of the gang of seven. A very potent combination of viral killers to help support your immune system.

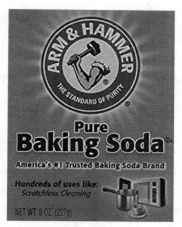

How to dose baking soda is simple (as outlined previously): You mix up a batch of it and you drink it on schedule. If done correctly, it could raise the pH of your body just enough to make it very difficult for the virus to spread through your body. Remember, you should begin taking baking soda by sipping it slowly to determine how your stomach is handling it. Never take it on a full stomach since it produces lots of gas, enough to potentially rupture your stomach! That could make for a really bad day.

OZONE

Since the advent of the COVID-19, practitioners from the medical underground all over the world have come up with ingenious, novel treatment strategies. The amazing ingenuity of many of those doctors is truly awe-inspiring. Many of these courageous doctors risk losing their medical licenses from state medical boards that are often unforgiving for doctors who are willing to think outside of the box to cure their patients by any means necessary.

One of those doctors on the front lines of treating COVID-19 is Dr. David Brownstein. Dr. Brownstein has a clinic outside of Detroit. He has been a pioneer in the use of iodine in medicine and has written many wonderful books that I encourage all of you to read.

With the outbreak of COVID-19, he once again pioneered a very effective treatment protocol. Of the 107 patients he and his team treated for COVID-19, he only had one hospitalization and no deaths! Early in the illness, he used the combination of hydrogen peroxide and iodine in nebulizer treatments. He almost immediately started vitamin C, vitamin A, and zinc. In addition to which, he used ozone to treat COVID-19.

Ozone chemically is O_3, or three oxygen atoms together. It is very unstable and breaks down to its more stable cousin O_2. Apparently, there are a number of ways to administer ozone, including intravenous, hyperbaric treatments and intramuscularly. However, you can use ozone-saturated carrier oils to deliver ozone to your body. It is especially useful in topical infections such as those on your skin, and I will discuss that further in the next chapter.

Ozone, vitamin C, and hydrogen peroxide all stimulate increased oxygen delivery to the cells of the body, either by their very nature or their increase in the body's production of hydrogen peroxide. Oxygen is deadly to many pathogens since many are anaerobes (thrive in an oxygen-free environment). It is also a known medical fact that wounds that do not bleed, do not heal. Blood flow equals oxygen delivery to tissues, which is essential for healing.

Alternative practitioners have pioneered the use of ozone from its humble beginning in the 1990s to the present day. Dr. Frank Shallenberger was one of the earliest pioneers of ozone therapy. Recently, Dr. David Brownstein has also had a lot of success treating various infections including COVID-19 with ozone.

Ozone is deadly upon contact to bacteria, fungi, parasites, and even viruses. It also stimulates the immune system to increase its production of infection fighting white blood cells, and thus antibodies, to kill any germs that are infecting us. Ozone also increases the production of what is known as reactive oxygen species, which are molecules that the body uses to kill deadly pathogens. In effect, ozone is involved in the direct release of oxygen into the body, which is known to kill almost all pathogens since they normally thrive in an anaerobic (without oxygen) environment.

Dr. Brownstein has been utilizing ozone in its various forms in his clinic in West Bloomfield, Michigan. He is way ahead of even most integrative and alternative practitioners in his use of ozone. He uses it in several forms including intravenous, intramuscular injection, and even in hyperbaric treatments. According to his experience, he has had great success in treating COVID-19 and other infections with ozone. Unfortunately for us, it is not widely available from doctors.

Dr. Robert Rowen is another physician who has developed significant expertise in the use of ozone. He first encountered it in Africa where he successfully treated Ebola patients with ozone therapy. He has a wonderful website for all things ozone called Ozone Without Borders. If you are interested in doing home ozone therapy, you can contribute twenty dollars, and he will send you a one-hour video that explains how to use this powerful technology at home. Unfortunately, it is beyond the scope of this book.

One thing to keep in mind is that ozone is deadly to lung tissue, and so it can never be inhaled in any form. For that reason, I am very reluctant to recommend it for home use. There are ozone generators available for the general public. However, its generation requires compressed medical grade oxygen along with the ozone generator. Sometimes, oxygen in this form is not available to the general public. You can also use an oxygen concentrator instead of the compressed medical-grade oxygen.

MELATONIN

Melatonin is a hormone produced by the pineal gland in the brain. It is widely known as a sleep aid to the general public, and it works very well in that role. What is not widely known is the widespread beneficial effects of melatonin on the body as a whole.

One hint to melatonin's usefulness is its presence in the earliest life-forms, unicellular or single-cell life-forms, in Earth's primordial soup. It has stayed with us all through our evolution, and that is not by chance. When nature develops a useful substance like melatonin, it wisely uses it over and over again all through various life-forms all the way up to man.

Melatonin is important for sleep, and its production is very sensitive to ambient (your surroundings) light levels. Even a night-light on in your bedroom can diminish your melatonin production. Conversely during the day, being exposed to bright light helps suppress melatonin production, saving it for greater release that evening in the dark.

Unfortunately, these days, we sit in front of our computer screens for hours on end indoors. Nothing could be worse for melatonin production since blue light from computers and LED light bulbs are some of the greatest inhibitors of melatonin production.

Remember, I always recommend lots of rest, hydration, and a good uninterrupted night's sleep as the very first step to take in treating any infection.

Melatonin is a very potent antioxidant and, as such, is critically important in the protection of your mitochondria, which are the energy producers for your cells. If mitochondria get damaged by oxidation, you will have a significant drop-off in your energy levels. That is why deep, uninterrupted sleep in a dark room is so critical to your health.

Melatonin actually enters into the mitochondria and protects them and also helps generate large amounts of glutathione, which as you remember from earlier in this book is essential to the proper immune function.

As an antioxidant, melatonin is more powerful than vitamins C, E, and even the very powerful glutathione, which it helps recharge as well.

Melatonin is also a potent antioxidant and anti-inflammatory hormone. As such, it is very useful in COVID-19 in the squelching of the body's out-of-control immune response that results in what is known as a *cytokine storm*. This exaggerated immune response is what causes the deadly cytokine storm, which is responsible for so many deaths from COVID-19.

Melatonin works synergistically (they support each other's actions) with vitamin D3, meaning the two are much more powerful together than each individually. For our purposes, vitamin D3 is already on board since we started our treatment protocol with our "gang of seven."

There is no set dose of melatonin. I personally take 10 mg every night, and I try to go to bed well before midnight since the healthiest schedule is to follow nature as closely as possible. Meaning going to sleep when the sun sets and getting up with sunrise and getting outside into that health-enhancing sunlight as much as your skin tone can take without burning.

I have to say, melatonin does give you vivid dreams since you go into such a deep level of sleep. I actually like it, finding my dreams to be immensely entertaining. Many mornings, I awake with vivid recollections of my nighttime forays into my dreamscape wonderland. If you have COVID-19, take up to 40 mg; it really has no side effects other than a deep sleep, which as I have mentioned is immensely useful for you.

IVERMECTIN

Last, but not least, is the use of ivermectin in the treatment of COVID-19. The goal of this book is to teach you all ways to treat infections primarily without the use of prescription medications. However, since ivermectin is so effective against most viral infections including COVID-19, I felt it would be remiss of me not to include it in the prevention and treatment sections of this chapter. As I stated earlier in this chapter when discussing the use of ivermectin in the prevention of COVID-19, the most experienced group in the world is the FLCCC.

The FLCCC treatment protocol has many components including treatment with ivermectin. The doses they recommend are 0.4 to 0.6 mg per kilogram of body weight daily. For most patients, this works out to three 12 mg tablets daily. It should be taken with food for better absorption. For a mild illness, it should be taken for five consecutive days. For a serious illness, it should be taken until you have recovered.

So, there you have it, the most potent treatments for COVID-19 currently available without a prescription, all readily available to you. You start with the "gang of seven" and your nebulizer treatments and layer in the other treatments at your preference. As I said, there is no known cure for COVID-19, but I have given you the best options for both prevention and treatment, which have arisen from the medical underground.

One last thought on COVID-19 and the current pandemic. Like the flu, coronaviruses have an animal reservoir. In flu, the reservoir is in wild birds; in coronaviruses, it is in bats. For that reason, it will never be eradicated, just like the flu. We have always had coronaviruses and always will. COVID-19 has been weaponized to a certain degree by Dr. Anthony Fauci and his diabolical colleagues by way of "gain of function" experiments that have increased its affinity for your respiratory system.

Currently, the thousands of variants that are arising are overwhelmingly from the vaccinated, where there is selective pressure on the virus to mutate in order to evade their immune systems. Viruses almost exclusively mutate into less lethal but more contagious versions of themselves. This satisfies the viruses' need to infect new hosts in order to survive. Keeping that trend in mind, it is relatively easy to foresee where this entire pandemic is heading. In my opinion, there will be an endless stream of variants arising, and each new wave will be progressively less lethal but ever more contagious. Eventually, the evolution of the virus will reach a point where the available "virgin" hosts are too few and far between to support a pandemic. That along with herd immunity from those previously infected, and to a lesser degree from those vaccinated, will result in it eventually petering out and ceasing to be a threat to our health or survival. Now that above scenario is what will happen to a virus "on its own," without the interference of mad scientists. The Chinese, Russians, Iranians, and North Koreans to name a few of our global adversaries have without a doubt noted how effective a bioweapon can be in devastating their enemies without one shot being fired. Sadly, but realistically I think we can expect many more pandemics in our future. This book will prove to be an invaluable source of information from the medical underground on how to prevent and treat any infection that may be unleashed upon us.

CHAPTER EIGHT

SKIN INFECTIONS

THE STRUCTURE OF HUMAN SKIN

The skin is composed of collagen embedded in a meshwork of other proteins. All the connective tissue in your body is made primarily of collagen, hence it is the most abundant protein in the human body. Collagen forms a network of fibers in the skin that give it structural support and are interwoven with elastic fibers that allow the skin to stretch.

There are also glycosaminoglycans, which store large amounts of water and keep the skin well hydrated, preventing it from drying out. The skin also contains sebaceous glands that secrete oils to keep skin well lubricated and pliable. There are three layers to the skin: the outer layer or epidermis, the middle layer or dermis, and the inner fat layer known as the subcutaneous layer or subcutis.

Collagen is essential for skin health. We used to have no problem with that because we ate animals like most of the world's people still do, from nose to tail. In between which there is lots of collagen—in animal skin, organs, and other various connective tissue elements.

Our current "modern diet" often includes skinless cuts of meat and very little animal organs and other animal parts that are high in collagen, hence it is severely lacking in collagen intake. That leaves most Americans the option of reverting to eating the entire animal or the need to supplement their collagen intake, usually with collagen powders. Call me crazy, but I think most Americans will not eat the entire animal.

Collagen powder works as long as you have adequate vitamin C, which is essential in its production. There are many types of collagen, and the best powder supplements contain a mix of different collagen types. I recommend that you take 5 grams of collagen powder daily for maintenance and increase that to three times a day for wound repair or any skin infections or conditions such as acne, eczema, or psoriasis.

Zinc is the other element your skin needs. If you are not supplementing with zinc, then you should start immediately. Just like vitamin C, zinc is not stored by the body, so you need to maintain your daily intake of both. Zinc and vitamin C are essential for DNA repair and collagen production. Zinc also has many other skin benefits. It is anti-inflammatory, antibacterial, antiviral, antiaging, and increases collagen synthesis and oil production by sebaceous glands to help lubricate and keep skin soft and supple.

Applied topically, zinc oxide is one of the best skin protectants. It reflects UV light and is inert, meaning it doesn't cause any problems for people who have very sensitive skin. I still remember all the lifeguards in the 1960s with zinc oxide smeared over their noses to prevent sunburns. Applied topically, zinc will lower your risk of skin cancer. A diet deficient in zinc will lead to acne, dermatitis, and eczema.

As with all nutrients, zinc is best obtained from food sources. Your body readily recognizes zinc in this form, and thus it is much better absorbed. Good food sources of zinc include beans, chicken, beef, cashews, chickpeas, and pumpkin seeds. My personal favorite food source of zinc is from oysters, in addition to which, they are purported to be an aphrodisiac! Talk about a great side effect! Let big pharma try to beat that one. Both selenium and niacin (vitamin B3) also increase zinc absorption.

Remember this: your skin as originally constructed required collagen, vitamin C, and zinc and a smattering of other proteins and minerals. All three are essential to form its final structure. Skin is constantly being produced by your body; therefore, we continually require all three just for our normal maintenance. Our body needs vastly more of all three when repairing skin from eczema, psoriasis, or acne, burns, infections, and tears from trauma.

SIGNS AND SYMPTOMS OF A SKIN INFECTION

The cardinal signs of a skin infection are red, warm, or hot skin, with or without a pustular discharge (pus oozing out of it) that may or may not be painful to touch. It may or may not be accompanied by a fever—usually it is not, unless there is blood borne spread (sepsis). Another sign of a wound infection is a foul smell. Either put your face down near the wound and sniff around, or if available, it is much easier to smell the wound dressing. You learn these things after decades "in the trenches."

Sepsis may also be accompanied by shaking chills (rigors), tremors, and there may be some confusion or delirium, especially in the elderly. Sepsis is usually accompanied by a fever greater than 101 degrees F; other times, the patient will be cold with a temp less than 95 degrees F.

Fever is usually accompanied by an increase in your pulse or heart rate. For each degree of fever, the pulse typically rises ten beats per minute. The baseline respiratory rate of approximately eighteen breaths per minute will often go into the twenties. Sepsis is a medical emergency and should be evaluated ASAP by a physician.

If you have dead-appearing black tissue, you have what is known as necrosis. This needs to be removed to allow healing. That is best done by someone who knows what they are doing such as a doctor, nurse, or physician's assistant.

Frequently, a skin or wound infection will spread to surrounding tissue. You want to know if that is happening. The best thing to do is to draw a line with a magic marker around the leading edge of the infection so in the ensuing days, you will be able to tell if it is spreading. The area around a wound will invariably become inflamed and oftentimes is painful to touch.

There may be inflamed lymph nodes draining the infected area. If for example the infection is on your face, on the same side of your neck, there will often be enlarged lymph nodes that will feel like small marbles.

A fungal infection is sometimes difficult to differentiate from a bacterial infection. Sometimes, you luck out and there are simply a bunch of rings with a red spreading edge and a blanched lighter central area. Fungal infections are often itchy; some like jock itch and athlete's foot are intensely itchy. By contrast, bacterial infections almost never itch.

TREATMENT OF SKIN INFECTIONS

BACTERIAL SKIN INFECTIONS

In the event of any skin infection, the first thing you should do is to either start or increase your intake of the three essential building blocks of skin production listed above: zinc, collagen, and vitamin C. Then I would suggest start taking the remaining members of the gang of seven in order to boost your immunity, which is universally helpful with any infection anywhere.

Any of the treatments listed below will help treat a skin infection, and several may be combined to further enhance their potency.

IODINE

Iodine, as I discussed in great detail in chapter 5, is an antiseptic and as such is extremely effective in killing all pathogens, including bacteria, viruses, and fungi. Iodine is also helpful in skin repair by helping to moisturize and regenerate it. These are the reasons that topical iodine should be the first thing you go to in the event of any skin infection.

You should always have a bottle of Betadine in your medicine cabinet for just such a problem. In the event of a skin infection, take a cotton ball or a four-by-four skin pad, soak it with a generous amount of Betadine, and apply it to your skin twice a day. Press the soaked cotton ball directly against the area you are treating and hold it there for ten seconds (count ten Mississippis if you are not sure).

For serious skin infections, allow it to soak in for up to two minutes. That will allow the iodine solution enough time to seep into the wound or infected area. It may give you a slight burning sensation, which is perfectly normal. It directly kills all pathogens on contact, and for this reason, even in these days of antibiotic resistance, it is still universally used in hospitals and other medical settings to sterilize skin and other surfaces. Iodine works so quickly that no bacterial resistance can develop. Betadine is readily available without a prescription in any pharmacy.

If you need to irrigate a deeper wound or infection, you could mix one part Betadine with nine parts of sterile water. This mix will allow you to flush out a deep nonsurface wound to either prevent or treat an infection.

Betadine or any other topical iodine preparation such as Lugol's solution, nascent iodine, tincture of iodine, and other liquid iodines should be kept away from the eyes since it may cause inflammation. If by chance it happens, flush them out with copious amounts of water.

Topical iodine solutions are not recommended for children under the age of one because the load of iodine is too strong for their young thyroid glands.

Iodine can also stain the skin an orange/brown color. If this occurs on your healthy skin, you can easily remove the stain with an alcohol pad. Skin reactions to topical iodine preparations are rare, but if the skin blisters or appears red and irritated, then immediately discontinue its use. The use of topical iodine is not recommended for deep puncture wounds or severe burns. The literature also discourages its use in animal bites, but I disagree. I have used it for years to clean animal bites with absolutely no problems.

HONEY

Any damage to the skin, be it an abrasion (scrape), tear (wound), or burn will benefit from the use of topical honey. Honey never spoils and thus has an indefinite shelf life, as long as you keep it covered to prevent it from drawing in too much water. The reason honey has such a great shelf life is due to its antibacterial, antifungal, and antiviral properties. Nothing can live in honey, so it never spoils. For our purposes, it is great to apply to any skin injury.

Among honeys, there is a hierarchy of potency with manuka honey being the most potent. Manuka honey comes from New Zealand and gets its name from the manuka bush from which local bees make it. It has wonderful wound-healing properties. However, that being said, any honey will work to keep a wound both well hydrated and free from infection.

Be generous when applying honey to a wound; fill up any holes and cover it completely. Then cover the honey with a double wound dressing of four-by-fours or whatever dressing material you have. When the outer dressing gets wet, that is your signal to reapply the honey and change the dressing.

Honey will not only keep the wound clean and moist but will also provide nourishment and improve healing. I have used it for decades in my practice, many times replacing unbelievably expensive "wound salves" with very good success. It is also something readily available and inexpensive that most patients already have in their pantries.

ALOE VERA

Aloe vera is also hugely helpful to healing damaged skin from burns, including sunburn. It will also soothe chaffed or abraded skin or raw exposed skin.

Aloe vera is mostly water, but it is also jam-packed with minerals, vitamins, amino acids, fatty acids and over two hundred active plant compounds that work wonders on healing and nourishing skin.

It is reported to have antibacterial and antiviral properties and will help prevent and treat minor skin infections. It does promote wound healing in two ways: by increasing collagen production and also by moisturizing the skin. This positive effect on the collagen not only helps skin heal but almost decreases scar formation.

There are several forms of aloe vera. I prefer the almost pure 99 percent or the pure 100 percent aloe vera gel. It is even available combined with tea tree oil or manuka honey, both of which add additional skin benefits. You could easily grow the plant and break off a leaf and split it open lengthwise and scoop out the healing gel and apply it directly to your skin.

The dose depends on the severity of the skin problem. If it is only chaffed skin, then once a day will suffice. More serious skin conditions including acne, burns, and superficial wounds would benefit from two- or three-times-a-day application. It is cooling and soothing to any irritated or burnt skin and feels great going on. I highly recommend it for any skin lesions.

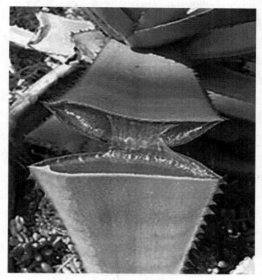

A split aloe vera leaf courtesy of Wikipedia

OZONE

Ozone is a great example of a very promising treatment that has been thoroughly vetted by the medical underground and virtually ignored by mainstream medicine.

Ozone's many uses are currently being explored by the medical underground and are slowly spreading to those of us "in the know."

What exactly is ozone? The oxygen we breathe is composed of two oxygen atoms; ozone is three oxygen atoms connected together. This molecule has some unique properties, one of which is it is ten times more soluble in water than the oxygen we breathe.

This is important because this allows ozone to dissolve in bodily fluids, especially human blood. Once it is dissolved in blood, it can be transported throughout the body and is easily absorbed by areas of the body that need it. Blood with ozone dissolved in it delivers much more oxygen than normal blood.

Lightning produces ozone by exposing atmospheric oxygen to an electrical charge, turning O_2 to O_3. Inside the body, O_3 ozone combines with other oxygen molecules and produces O_2 once again. This frees oxygen in the form of O_2 within the body.

Ozone (and oxygen) has the wonderful property of being deadly to bacteria, fungi, yeasts, parasites, and viruses. It kills all viruses on contact. It does this by using the free oxygen molecule that it releases in the body. This free oxygen scavenger goes around and tears holes in the walls of all pathogens, being universally deadly.

In addition to which, ozone is a strong stimulator of the immune system. It stimulates the body to vastly increase its production of white blood cells and antibodies. In fact, the genius Nikola Tesla was the inventor of the first ozone-generating machine around 1900.

Ozone, vitamin C, and hydrogen peroxide all stimulate increased oxygen delivery to the cells of the body. They do this directly by their very nature or indirectly by their stimulation of the body's production of hydrogen peroxide. Either way, they increase the delivery of oxygen in its various forms to the body.

For our purposes, ozone can be applied topically to treat skin infections. The ozone is infused into a carrier oil. A carrier oil is simply an oil that is used as a solvent, meaning the ozone dissolves into it and in that form, it easily penetrates the skin.

There are many varieties of ozonated carrier oils on the market, including coconut oil, safflower oil, grapeseed oil, and olive oil to name but a few. They will work to treat any skin infection, whether caused by bacteria, fungi, or viruses, since ozone is deadly to all of them.

DAKIN'S SOLUTION

During WWI, there was an overwhelming demand for methods to clean the wounds of the hundreds of thousands of wounded men who were dying in large numbers from infections. An American chemist named Harold Dakin went to England as a volunteer for their war effort. His contribution appropriately named Dakin's solution stays with us to this day, more than one hundred years later. It does so because it is easy to make and very effective at cleaning and disinfecting any wound to the skin.

HERE IS HOW YOU MAKE IT:

Take four cups or 32 ounces of sterilized water. You can easily sterilize water by boiling it for fifteen minutes in a covered pot.

Add one-half of a teaspoon of sodium bicarbonate (baking soda)

Now here is the tricky part: you add bleach (Clorox or regular household bleach), depending on the severity of the wound.

For clean wounds or dressing changes, add three teaspoons of bleach. If the wound is mildly infected, add three tablespoons of bleach. If severely infected, add three fluid ounces of bleach (95 ml).

For dressing changes, once a day will suffice; for all others, use it twice a day.

Note: A premade batch of this solution will not last longer than two days. Also, be aware that if you have old bleach lying around, it may have lost its potency. If you have no other option, double its concentration.

Note: If you are cleaning a dirty wound, try your best to remove any dirt or foreign objects from the wound before you irrigate it with Dakin's or other wound-cleansing solutions. Also, make sure you are either wearing gloves or have thoroughly cleansed your hands to disinfect them and avoid introducing new pathogens.

HERBAL WOUND-CLEANSING SOLUTIONS

Herbal wound cleansers can also be made using essential oils added to sterile water. There is no precise formula for this; just add a drop of liquid soap and a few drops of essential oil to the water and irrigate the wound with it. Be generous in the amount of either Dakin's solution or your herbal mix you use to clean the wound. The following essential oils are useful as wound cleansers: eucalyptus oil, lavender oil, rosemary oil, peppermint oil, and tea tree oil.

ACTIVATED CHARCOAL

Activated charcoal is very effective at both keeping a wound clean as well as promoting wound healing. Activated charcoal has been recognized for its antimicrobial effects since the time of ancient Egypt.

It not only is antimicrobial, but it is also an effective treatment for venomous bites of all types and is a powerful antitoxin, inactivating toxins of all types.

Activated charcoal is so amazingly effective due to its structure. It has an immense surface area, so large that if you were able to "unwind" one gram of activated charcoal, it would cover about a thousand square meters of surface area! It works its wonders not by absorption but rather adsorption.

Absorption acts like a sponge, with the absorbed material soaking into and swelling it. Adsorption is different; it works by electrostatically binding substances to its surface, thus inactivating it. It is so potent that one quart of activated charcoal will soak up 80 quarts of ammonia gas. If it was absorbing materials, it would swell to an incredible size, which is not the case. It does not swell at all, just chemically changing substances to inactivate them.

Activated charcoal is incredible for filtering water and has endless applications in our heavily polluted world. A great website that describes all things "charcoal" is CharcoalRemedies.com; it is full of fascinating information.

For our purposes, it is amazing wound cleaner and disinfectant. Let's take a look how to use it.

The best way to use activated charcoal on a wound is to make a poultice. A poultice is a soft, moist paste that is applied directly to a wound. The key word there is *moist*. If a poultice dries out, it loses its potency and is essentially worthless.

Activated charcoal poultices can be made two ways—either with straight activated charcoal or with the addition of flaxseed. I prefer the combination with flaxseed since it both thickens it and helps it retain moisture.

HERE IS HOW TO MAKE YOUR FLAXSEED/ ACTIVATED CHARCOAL POULTICE:

Grind three tablespoons of flaxseed (alternatively you can use cornstarch).

Add two or three tablespoons of activated charcoal powder.

Add one cup of water you can add more or less, depending upon how thick you want your poultice.

Stir them together well and allow the mix to sit for fifteen minutes to thoroughly combine. Alternatively, you can put it into a pot and gently heat it to help facilitate the mixing.

Spread the poultice mix onto a clean cloth and apply directly to the wound, making sure you have good contact between the two.

Cover the first dressing with a dry clean dressing.

Wrap the entire dressing with a plastic covering, such as a plastic bag or plastic food wrap. Make sure you overlap the sides of the underlying cloth dressing by an inch or so on either side. Then use surgical tape, or if you don't have that, duct tape will work just fine. This step is critical. If you don't tape the sides well, air will get into the poultice and prematurely dry it out, thus rendering it ineffective. It is important to take the time to do it right.

Leave the poultice on the wound and change it whenever it dries out or daily. The poultice will also act as a mechanical barrier, protecting the involved area of skin and keeping it clean of foreign debris.

Note: This poultice will work for any burn, bites of any kind including spiders, snakes, and scorpions. It will also help soothe a bad poison ivy, poison oak, or poison sumac rash.

TEA TREE OIL

Tea tree oil, also known as melaleuca, is an essential oil made from steaming the leaves of the Australian tea tree. It has wonderful antimicrobial effects, treating both bacterial and fungal infections. It may even be beneficial in the treatment of MRSA, although that remains somewhat controversial. It works very well against fungal infections of the skin such as jock itch and athlete's foot.

Tea tree oil is poisonous if ingested and should never be taken internally or used near the mouth where some may be inadvertently swallowed.

Tea tree oil may be used full strength on intact skin but, on broken skin, should be diluted to a 10 percent solution. That basically means one part tea tree oil to nine parts of the dilutant. It can be diluted with a variety of substances including water, aloe, olive oil, macadamia nut oil, safflower oil, eucalyptus oil, lavender oil, or rose geranium oil.

Full-strength tea tree oil may cause burning and even blistering in sensitive skin. It is available as a topical antiseptic ointment already diluted to its proper strength. It should be applied two or three times a day, depending on the severity of the infection.

To treat a fungal skin infection, use a 50 percent solution of tea tree oil—for those of you who are math challenged, that means half tea tree oil and half dilutant.

HYDROGEN PEROXIDE

Hydrogen peroxide is a very effective and inexpensive wound and skin cleanser and antiseptic. It is readily available in its most common 3 percent form in any pharmacy or convenience store. Hydrogen peroxides chemical formula is H_2O_2; when it breaks down, it breaks down to water and oxygen. Oxygen, as we have previously discussed, is a very potent antimicrobial.

Some medical sites warn of the dangers of straight hydrogen peroxide on skin. For short-term use, I have never seen even one adverse reaction in my more than thirty-seven years of clinical practice. Long term, it may dry out skin excessively and even cause some redness and irritation.

The reality is we are not using it except to either disinfect some skin or to treat an existing infection, so use it full strength with no worries. If you do, by chance, develop some reddening of the skin or irritation, dilute it with some saline solution or water. If it persists, then discontinue its use.

It is sad that I have to say that. It is like the warning on ladders: "Do not go above top step it may be dangerous." You see, I am of a contrary school of thought that states, "Maybe… just maybe, natural selection exists for a very good reason." Nature rarely, if ever, makes mistakes.

Contrary to most patients' opinions, it does not burn a wound when applied (they confuse it with topical alcohol), nor does it have a smell. For years, countless times I have opened bottles of hydrogen peroxide and placed it under the noses of my patients, almost universally, they cringe and scrunch up their noses in anticipation of it stinking. I do that to demonstrate that it has no smell and no taste, knowing that if I didn't do that, no matter what I say, most will not try it.

As I said earlier, the most common form of hydrogen peroxide is the 3 percent dilution found in most stores. Studies have shown that at this strength, it is deadly to bacteria, viruses, and even fungal infections. It also helps when applied to wounds to chemically debride it by loosening up clots and dirt as it "foams up" the dirty wound.

Some report that it may be too strong and actually damage healthy cells around the wound edges. I have not found that to be the case in my extensive experience in clinical practice. If used short term, that is for two weeks or less, I have never seen any skin damage from hydrogen peroxide.

Reports of skin bleaching are not from the 3 percent, but from much stronger strengths of hydrogen peroxide typically available online. I do not recommend using any higher strength; there is absolutely no need for it. For the purposes of wound disinfection, there is no need to get "food grade" hydrogen peroxide. That is preferable only for internal use such as in a nebulizer.

The way to use hydrogen peroxide for any infected wounds or skin is to take a few cotton balls or a small four-by-four gauze and soak them and apply them directly to the wound or infection site. Leave them on for a few seconds and remove them. You will notice the area foaming up as the bacteria and other microbes are killed by the peroxide. That is a good thing. Don't worry, it will not burn or sting in the least.

If there is a gaping wound that you are worried about becoming infected or if you feel it is already infected, then pour a small amount of hydrogen peroxide directly into the wound. Do it two or three times a day, depending upon the severity of the infection.

FUNGAL SKIN INFECTIONS

The most common fungal skin infections are jock itch (fungal infection of the groin area, applies to females as well as males), athlete's foot, ringworm, and other fungal skin infections. Often, the obese will have fungal infections in their abdominal folds due to the area being warm and sweaty, a perfect environment for a fungal infection to flourish. The good news is that no matter where the fungal infection is located, they are all treated the same.

SYMPTOMS OF A FUNGAL RASH

Depending upon the location, fungal rashes appear differently. For example, ringworm will look like red rings with a lighter-color center. These typically appear on the arms, face, legs, and torso. Ringworm is highly contagious. Jock itch will be in the groin and often spreads to the insides of the thighs and around into the perianal area (the area around the anus or your butthole).

Jock itch will be red and often warm and, many times, will have a red spreading edge to it. Athlete's foot will involve peeling, cracked red skin on the soles of the feet and heels. Other times, it is a white area between the toes, with or without skin cracking and peeling. It is usually intensely itchy.

TREATMENT OF FUNGAL SKIN INFECTIONS

IODINE

My first go-to treatment for fungal skin infections of all kinds is iodine. Iodine is lethal to all fungal infections, bacteria, and viruses. It is inexpensive and readily available. You can either use Betadine, Lugol's solution, nascent iodine, or any other form of liquid iodine. Apply it to a gauze pad or a few cotton balls and apply it to the skin infection; leave it on it for two minutes.

Studies have shown that after ninety-plus seconds, the vast majority of bacteria, fungi, and yeast infections are killed by iodine. If it is a serious fungal infection, do these two or three times a day until healed.

Another area of fungal infection that is many times quite resistant to treatment is when toenails (and fingernails to a much lesser degree) are yellowed, thick, and crusty. Studies have shown that painting toenails twice a day with Betadine will safely and effectively eradicate those very-hard-to-treat infections. Keep in mind that it takes twelve to eighteen months for an entire toenail like the big toe to grow out normally.

TEA TREE OIL

Tea tree oil is readily available in most pharmacies and works against all kinds of skin infections, including fungal.

To treat a fungal skin infection, use a 50 percent solution of tea tree oil. For those of you who are math challenged, that means half tea tree oil and half dilutant. I described earlier in this chapter how to dilute tea tree oil.

Probably the best dilutant is coconut oil since it contains medium-chain triglycerides that also have antifungal activity. In addition, coconut oil contains caprylic acid that kills yeast by perforating their cell wall without damaging normal cells.

Apply it two or three times a day until healed. If any irritation of the healthy skin appears to be occurring, then dilute it down to one quarter strength.

There are other essential oils that also have antifungal properties, such as eucalyptus, geranium, patchouli, myrrh, and lavender oils. But none are as effective as tea tree oil.

APPLE CIDER VINEGAR

Apple cider vinegar (ACV) also has antifungal properties and is good for treating fungal skin infections. By far, the best apple cider vinegar to use for fungal skin infections is the raw, unprocessed, and unfiltered type such as the brand Bragg, which is readily available in grocery stores.

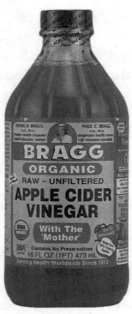

ACV contains acetic acid, which is the active ingredient in it that is fungicidal (kills fungus). In its raw form, it contains many enzymes that also help in its antifungal role.

Apple cider vinegar should be diluted 50/50 with water. Full strength may irritate the skin a little. However, that being said, if you have a really bad, kick-ass fungal infection, you might want to go full strength for the first couple of applications then reduce it to half strength.

ACV compresses can be made by soaking a facecloth in apple cider vinegar and then gently squeezing out the excess. Apply that directly to the fungal skin infection and leave it on for fifteen minutes then allow it to air-dry. Do this two or three times a day until it is healed.

Conversely, you can soak a gauze pad or some cotton balls into your mixture and apply it generously to the fungal infection twice a day then allow to air-dry.

If you have a widespread fungal skin infection, you can soak in a bath of ACV and lukewarm water. Depending upon how severe your infection is, use between six and eight cups of ACV in your bathwater. Immerse yourself in this ACV-water mix for about twenty minutes. Do this nightly until you are healed.

BORAX

Borax, yes, the same thing as the laundry detergent famous for its twenty-mule teams turns out to be a strong antifungal. It also has many other beneficial health properties, especially for osteopenia and osteoporosis that I use it extensively in my practice. Borax contains boric acid, which is made up mostly of the mineral boron. You can either use Borax laundry detergent or you can also buy boric acid online.

Borax laundry detergent (one cup) can be mixed in a bucket of warm water. Immerse your affected foot in it for about fifteen minutes daily and dry well when you remove them. You can also sprinkle some borax into your socks for mild athlete's foot. Alternatively, you can mix borax with some water and make a paste that you can rub into your fungal skin infections two or three times a day until healed.

When using boric acid, take two teaspoons of it and mix it thoroughly in one cup of water or rubbing alcohol. Soak cotton balls or gauze into the solution and apply two or three times daily to the infected area. You can also sprinkle some boric acid into your socks daily for a mild infection or for recurrent athlete's foot.

CHAPTER NINE

INFECTIONS OF THE GENITOURINARY TRACT:

BLADDER, KIDNEYS, VAGINA, AND PENIS

Let's first take a look at the anatomy of the genitourinary tract, so you better understand the pathology. First, we will take a look at the urinary tract, which includes your kidneys, ureters, bladder, and urethra.

The urinary tract also has two sets of muscles that control the sphincter at the exit from your bladder. The internal set of these sphincter muscles is involuntary (meaning you have no conscious control of them, your body does it for you).

The external set of sphincter muscles is voluntary, and you can consciously squeeze them to prevent you from urinating. Those are the muscles you use when, for example, you are someplace where you cannot urinate but need to, so you consciously squeeze them to wait until you get to a bathroom.

As you know, the kidneys are responsible for filtering the blood and removing anything the body can use, such as electrolytes, proteins, and sugar and excreting the remainder of its filtrate as urine. Ideally, your urine should be light yellow. If it is darker, it usually means that you are not adequately hydrated, and as a consequence, your urine is more concentrated.

Hydration is of paramount importance for your overall health and especially for your renal (kidney) health. The reason for that is that if you are not well hydrated, your blood volume will contract; less blood is delivered to your kidneys for filtration.

Your kidneys filter between 120 and 150 quarts of blood daily, producing one to two liters of urine on average. If your state of dehydration is chronic, it will impair your body from excreting its waste products and impair renal filtration of your blood. You see, as your body goes through its day-to-day function, it naturally produces lots of waste products.

Most of the waste is water soluble, meaning it dissolves in water and thus enters your blood and is delivered to the kidneys for filtration and excretion in your urine. Your kidneys will also excrete excess fluid, so you are not fluid overloaded, for example. That is why you pee like a racehorse when you drink too much beer. This prevents your body form being flooded with excess amounts of water, and just as important, it gives your friends something to goof on you about.

Urinary Tract

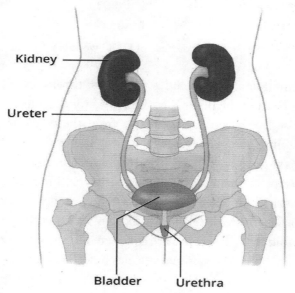

Kidney

Ureter

Bladder   Urethra

The genital tracts of women are composed of external vulva, a vagina, a uterus above the vagina, connected to it by a cervix. The uterus is connected above by two fallopian tubes (also called oviducts), which transport the monthly ovum or egg from the ovaries to the uterus. The infections that we will be addressing later on in this chapter include vaginal bacterial and yeast infections, external yeast infections of the vulva, urethral infections. Bladder infections and venereal infections

Female anatomy

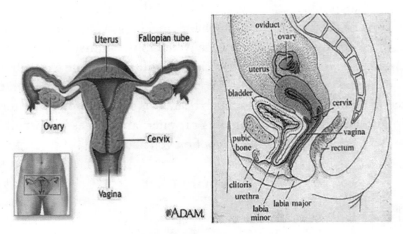

Drawing courtesy of CDC website.

Male genital anatomy includes the penis, through which runs the urethra. The head of the penis is covered by a foreskin in those who are not circumcised. Proceeding backwards from the penis into the body, we find the following:

At the base of the penis the urethra passes through the doughnut-shaped prostate and continues on into the bladder. The bladder is connected to the kidneys by the ureters. The testicles are contained in the scrotum. The testes itself looks like an acorn with the acorn cap being the epididymis. The testes are connected to the urethra via the vas deferens, which joins the seminal vesicles before doing so.

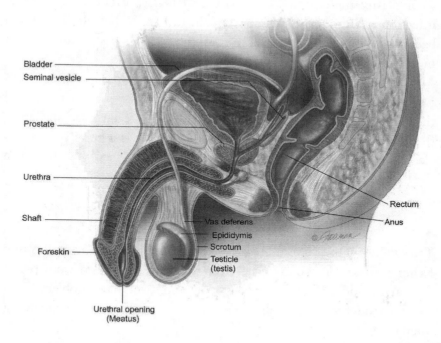

Drawing courtesy of the Urological Care Foundation.

The male genital infections that we will be addressing later on in this chapter include urethral infections, bladder infections, venereal infections, and epididymitis.

PREVENTION OF URINARY TRACT INFECTIONS (UTIS)

Emptying your bladder periodically will help keep your bladder muscles tight and functioning properly. If you habitually retain urine for long periods of time, it has the effect of weakening your bladder wall.

Also, when you retain urine in your bladder, it becomes a petri dish for the growth of bad bacteria, which leads to urinary tract infections. This is why hydration is so important since it will produce more urine and therefore increase your urination. That increased urinary flow will flush out your kidneys, ureters, bladder, and urethra, preventing infections.

Healthy bathroom habits will also help prevent urinary tract infections. After sex, it is important to urinate to help flush out any bacteria that may have entered your urethra. This is important for both men and women.

Women should also wipe themselves after a bowel movement from front to back. This will prevent depositing fecal bacteria at the front of the urethra, leading to a bladder infection. If you are a woman and suffer from frequent urinary tract infections (UTIs), it is a good practice to clean your genital area both before and after sex. This will greatly reduce the bacteria present and thus prevent many infections.

KEGEL EXERCISES

You can help improve your bladder strength and function by performing Kegel exercises. These exercises strengthen the muscles of your pelvic floor and bladder. They are simple to do, and if you have problems with a weak bladder or incontinence (leaking urine), then I recommend doing them several times a day.

Here is how you do them:

1. For both men and women, imagine you are trying to prevent passing gas, consciously squeezing your anus closed. As you do so, you will feel a pulling sensation as those muscles appropriately tighten. Do a set of these ten times in a row, three times daily. Hold the muscles tight for a count of three, then relax for a count of three and repeat.

2. For women, imagine you are sitting on a marble and trying to pick it up with your vagina, sucking it in. Next, lie down and slide a finger into your vagina, now squeeze as if you are trying to stop urine from leaking out. Once again, hold for a count of three and then relax for a count of three and repeat. Do this three times a day.

If done properly, you should feel your pelvic muscles tightening on your finger. Do both of these for a set of ten, three sets a day. If done properly, this will greatly help to strengthen your vaginal and bladder muscles and help with any problems with urgency and incontinence.

It will also tighten your vagina. When performing your Kegel exercises, do not tighten other sets of muscles such as your abdominal or leg muscles. This may put too much pressure on your bladder and be counterproductive.

OTHER WAYS TO PREVENT UTIS

There are some other simple strategies you can employ to prevent UTIs:

Drink lots of fresh water. Hydration is still king when trying to prevent UTIs. Nothing works as well as fresh water. Every "authority" says eight glasses a day, that is minimum. The more water, the better to flush out your urinary tract. Since most urinary tract infections are from outside sources such as feces, frequent drinking of copious amounts of water will help flush out the invaders.

Wipe yourself from front to back.

Acidify your urine by taking vitamin C daily. This will make your urine less receptive to bacteria by lowering the pH. I would recommend 1,000 mg (one gram) of time-release vitamin C once daily. If you have a severe problem with recurrent UTIs, then do it twice daily.

Squeezing fresh lemons into water will also help. Use a whole lemon over the course of a day in divided doses. Lemon juice has additional health benefits, such as promoting weight loss, boosting your immunity via its vitamin C content, aids in digestion, prevents calcium oxalate kidney stones (which are the most common), and contributes to your overall hydration.

Wear clean cotton underwear. This will allow proper air circulation and will prevent excess moisture from building up.

Clean your genital area before and after sex, especially around your urethral opening.

URINATE AFTER SEX

Drink unsweetened cranberry juice, which contains phenolic acids and antioxidants that prevent bacteria from adhering to the bladder wall. If you don't like cranberry juice or prefer to take it in capsule form, there are cranberry powder capsules that do the same thing. The typical dose is 500 mg one a day for prevention. As an aside, I recently discovered the wonderful combination of cranberry juice and lime—amazingly refreshing drink.

Use tampons instead of sanitary pads and change them every four to six hours.

After swimming, do not hang around in a wet bathing suit and dry yourself well, especially your genital area.

Women, if you masturbate, make sure your hands are cleansed beforehand with soap and water. If you are using sex toys of any type, make sure they are clean as well. You can immerse them in a 50 percent mix of water and hydrogen peroxide (for those of you who are math challenged, that means half water, half hydrogen peroxide). Soak them in that solution for fifteen minutes; dry it well, and you are all set.

Avoid the use of spermicides. These may cause irritation and may make it easier for bad bacteria to flourish.

Avoid the use of unlubricated condoms since the friction may cause irritation and cell damage, which can facilitate bacterial infections.

Women are more prone to UTIs for several reasons, including the nature of sex, with their genitalia being manually manipulated as well as male genital insertion. That is why it is important for her lover to make sure his hands are washed with soap and water before sex as well as the importance of urinating after sex.

It is also important for men to clean their penises after sex, especially if they are uncircumcised. There are also anatomical reasons for the prevalence of UTIs among women. Women have a very short distance between their urethral opening and their bladder, and their urethral opening is close to their rectum.

In men, depending on how lucky they are, the length of their penis is a considerable distance and a formidable barrier for microscopic bacteria to cross to reach their bladders. Did you ever wonder why men tend to name their penises and women almost never name their vaginas? I imagine it is one of those imponderable differences between the sexes. Vive la difference! However, I digress. Let's get back to the subject at hand.

PREVENTION OF VAGINAL INFECTIONS

The methods to prevent urinary tract infections are almost identical to those for vaginal infections, except for a few additions. Safe sexual practices and use of condoms, avoiding multiple sex partners, which increases your chances of coming across someone who is infected.

A big one is avoiding douching. This kills off the resident lactobacillus flora of the vagina and allows competing microorganisms to colonize the vagina and lead to infection. The only exception to the above rule about avoiding douching is the use of Betadine douches, which you will learn about later in this chapter.

Try to avoid scented feminine products and change tampons and feminine pads and panty liners frequently. And last but not least, avoid tight panties, jeans, and leggings, which look great but limit airflow.

PREVENTION OF HERPES INFECTIONS

The herpes virus family has an Achilles' heel that we can exploit to prevent them and also to treat them after an outbreak. Its vulnerability is the fact that the herpes virus requires the amino acid arginine to reproduce. The receptor on the cell surface has a special shape that matches arginine; it also matches another amino acid called L-lysine.

What I do with my patients who either have recurrent herpes infections (of any type) or a current outbreak is to put them on high-dose L-lysine tablets (500 mg three times a day with food), along with vitamin C (500 mg three times a day) to help boost their immune system.

You see, herpes infections are like an immune system seesaw. When the immune system is down, the herpes virus flourishes and starts reproducing unchecked. This produces the symptoms of burning before the outbreak, and then it reaches the skin, and lesions develop.

At any time either before or during an infection, you can flood your body with L-lysine and vitamin C and squelch the outbreak by preventing the virus from reproducing as well as boosting the immune system.

Note: The above prevention of genital herpes will work for any of the other herpes family infections including herpes labialis (herpes outbreak on your lips what are commonly called cold sores), and herpes zoster or shingles. It will also work for varicella zoster or what is commonly known as chicken pox; however, for children you will have to cut the doses in half. I am referring to young children, not infants. In the case of infants, you should consult your pediatrician.

SYMPTOMS OF GENITOURINARY TRACT INFECTIONS

Urinary tract infections (UTIs) primarily involve the bladder (cystitis) more than the urethra, ureters, and kidneys. UTIs manifest with symptoms of frequent urination, nocturia (getting up from sleep to urinate), dysuria (burning or painful urination). UTIs are sometimes accompanied by a fever, but it is not usually the case.

Women get urinary tract infections much more than men, usually as a contamination of their urinary tract from fecal bacteria. That is why it is so important for women to wipe themselves from front to back, not vice versa. Forty to sixty percent of women will suffer with a UTI sometime during their lives. An unfortunate 25 percent of women will suffer with recurrent UTIs.

Men get UTIs to a much lesser degree, and if they do, it usually involves some type of urinary tract obstruction, usually as a consequence of an enlarged prostate or from kidney stones. Men often get sexually transmitted infections, especially of their urethra, resulting in a painful penis with burning upon urination, oftentimes with a pustular discharge. Many times, the urethra is irritated from rough or prolonged sex. This will mimic a UTI with burning and a sensitive penis, but without fever or any discharge.

Any bladder infection can travel up to the kidneys and cause a kidney infection. This is a much more serious problem and will require antibiotics. It is more likely to happen to diabetics, immunocompromised patients, and those who are pregnant. These patients will be much sicker than a simple bladder infection. They often have high fevers, pus or blood in urine, abdominal pain, no appetite, cloudy or even fish-smelling urine, and severe pain upon urination.

Another area that can become infected is the urethra. This is known as urethritis. Its cardinal sign is painful urination, with or without a pustular discharge. Oftentimes, there is frequent urination, a bloody discharge, painful sex, and possibly lower abdominal pain. This can occur in both men and women.

For men, it is easily noted due to the length of their urethras and the fact that anything that affects a man's penis will immediately get his undivided attention. Men who routinely ignore crushing chest pain and shortness of breath will rush to my office with the first sign of a penis problem. We are who we are.

SYMPTOMS OF VAGINAL INFECTIONS

The vagina typically has three types of infections: bacterial, yeast or fungal, and parasitic from trichomoniasis. The symptoms overlap between them but usually include painful intercourse, with or without a vaginal discharge, and a raw painful vulva (external vaginal area). Any combination of the above spells a vaginal infection.

Bacterial infections usually are the result of a dysbiosis, meaning an abnormal bacterial overgrowth, thus displacing the normal flora of the vagina, which is lactobacillus. The new bacteria drive out the lactobacillus colonizing its territory in the vagina, shortly thereafter producing symptoms of an infection.

What causes this pathologic bacterial overgrowth? There are many causes including multiple sex partners, unsafe sexual practices, frequent douching, an IUD (intrauterine device), and even pregnancy.

The symptoms of a bacterial vaginitis are first and foremost a fishy-smelling, slimy vaginal discharge. The same kind of fishy discharge also occurs in trichomoniasis infections. This vaginitis causes burning upon urination and a discharge that is usually white or gray.

The discharge is not thick like cottage cheese but rather more like a slimy liquid. The vagina is usually somewhat irritated and may or may not be itchy. Sex is usually painful, but not always.

Yeast infections of the vagina are very common and, 75 percent of women get one or more during their lifetimes. These yeast infections typically occur after puberty and before menopause due to hormonal changes in the body that lead to changing conditions within the vagina. The flora of the vagina contains good yeast as well as good bacteria.

The good yeast is named candida. It has various subtypes, and the most common culprit for vaginal yeast infections is *Candida albicans*. It is the same species of yeast that colonizes the mouth (also the throat and gut), and when it takes over the mouth, you have what is known as thrush; in the vagina, it is *Candida vaginitis*.

As you can see, *Candida a.* has a dark side. Normally they are non-disease-causing members of our body's flora or microbiome. When our immune system is no longer capable of keeping it in check, it will explode in growth and cause thrush in our mouth and throat and vaginal yeast infections, among others. In cases of severe immune suppression, it can spread in our blood (sepsis), and in some cases even be fatal.

The main symptom that typically occurs is a thick clumpy white discharge similar in appearance to cottage cheese. The discharge typically does not smell bad, like bacterial vaginitis does. If you see a cottage cheese discharge, you have a yeast infection, plain and simple.

Other symptoms include sore vagina, painful sexual intercourse (not that frequent of a symptom), and itchiness to the vagina and external labia (external vaginal lips). In addition to which you may or may not have some discomfort upon urination.

Causes that lead to vaginal yeast infections include those that disrupt the normal pH of the vagina and hence the balance of normal vaginal flora (the good bacteria and yeast). Some causes are normal menses, recent antibiotic use (this once again disrupts the normal flora), pregnancy, diabetes (sugar feeds yeast), and even some contraceptives. In addition to which, anything that impairs the normal activity of the immune system could wind up with an overgrowth of yeast.

If you have diabetes, prevention is difficult, but nothing will do more than maintaining tight control of your blood glucose levels. Avoid antibiotic use as much as possible since they are often mistakenly prescribed for viral infections, for which they are totally useless.

Trichomoniasis is caused by a parasite aptly named trichomonas vaginalis. It is the most common sexually transmitted infection, probably because many times, it is asymptomatic (meaning they have no symptoms), so patients continue to have sex, not knowing they are infected. Another problem is the incubation period between exposure and actual symptoms, which is from five days to almost a month.

One of the symptoms that makes the diagnosis problematic is the fishy-smelling discharge since it also occurs in bacterial vaginitis. Just like both of the other causes of vaginitis, women often have painful intercourse; burning or itching feeling; red, sore genitals; and painful urination. None of which are specific for trichomoniasis. Keep in mind that the vast majority of women are asymptomatic.

SYMPTOMS OF A HERPES OUTBREAK

Unusual symptoms of infection are clear painful small blisters singly or in clusters. This is almost always a sign or symptom of an infection with herpes simplex virus or what is commonly known as herpes. It is easily spread because of its contagious nature and the fact that two-thirds of patients have little or no symptoms.

The same vesicles may or may not come back. The more often they recur, obviously, the worse for you. Oftentimes, they break open and form shallow painful ulcers that may become secondarily infected by bacteria. Sometimes, herpes infections just produce red bumps that may or may not be painful.

Oftentimes, there are prodromal symptoms, meaning warning symptoms, such as burning or tingling in the area before the lesions come out or very sensitive skin in the area of the future outbreak. Note, herpes recurs in the same location.

You see, herpes infections are like an immune system seesaw. When the immune system is down, the herpes virus is no longer controlled, and it flourishes and starts reproducing unchecked. This produces the symptoms of burning before the outbreak, and then it reaches the skin, and lesions develop.

At any time either before or during an infection, you can flood your body with L-lysine and vitamin C and squelch the outbreak by preventing the virus from reproducing as well as boosting the immune system. As I explained earlier in this chapter, the L-lysine will flood and occupy the arginine receptors and prevent the herpes virus from replicating. The amount of vitamin C you take depends.

If you are not on it, I would suggest to take minimum 500 mg with each L-lysine dose. If you are already on vitamin C, double your dose, for a minimum of one gram (1,000 mg) three times a day. By the way, any other immune-boosting vitamins and minerals will help suppress the viral outbreak as well.

Note: Everyone has heard the old joke, "What is the difference between love and herpes?" Answer, "Herpes is forever." As with all humor, it is based in truth. We have no cure for the herpes virus. Between outbreaks, it is stored in the nerves supplying the skin where the outbreak occurs.

Medically, that area of skin is known as a dermatome. That is why herpes outbreaks always return in the same area or dermatome; it is not a blood-borne infection. You should also note that herpes infections are very contagious before and during an outbreak, not in between. An outbreak of herpes can be spread from its original area on the lips, mouth to the genitals by oral sex, and vice versa.

SYMPTOMS OF VENEREAL DISEASES

One of the most common signs of a venereal disease is a painless round lump in the genital area. It can also be found around the anus, depending upon what kind of sex you had. In gay men, this is a commonly involved area. A pustular discharge from the penis or vaginal area is another sign. A rash may appear on the soles or palms or any other area.

There oftentimes are enlarged lymph nodes draining the infected area. Painful urination for both sexes, and for women, painful intercourse with or without a vaginal discharge is a possible symptom of a venereal disease.

There are many types of venereal diseases including condyloma acuminatum, gonorrhea, syphilis, chlamydia, HIV, trichomoniasis, and genital herpes. Many of the symptoms overlap. If you have had unprotected sex and think you have any one of these, you should be seen immediately by a physician. Also, refrain from having sex—you won't enjoy it anyway. And even with a condom, accidents can happen. It is totally selfish and unfair of you to risk infecting your partner.

Women should also keep in mind that if a venereal disease is left untreated, you may become infertile. Or if you do get pregnant, you can easily pass it to your newborn as it passes through the birth canal.

Not all the abovenamed venereal diseases carry symptoms. Some, like syphilis, have such mild initial symptoms that it oftentimes goes unnoticed or is mistaken for something else. Syphilis is known as the great imitator since it has such a variety of usually mild symptoms.

Left untreated, a chronic syphilis infection can cause horrendous damage to your health. Late-stage syphilis is also known as tertiary syphilis and can cause damage to the brain, blood vessels, nervous system, eyes, heart, and liver.

A relatively easy infection to identify is condyloma acuminatum or genital or venereal warts. It is easy because in men, the warts are readily evident. In women, if intravaginal, it is harder to spot. Sometimes they are located outside the vagina; naturally, this is easy to spot. It is caused by human papillomavirus (HPV). It is one of the most common venereal diseases.

We don't have many options for treating symptoms of these other than short-term boosting the immune system for example from the "gang of seven." Any rashes or lesions on the outside can be treated like any other skin infection, but that is a temporary fix and will not address the potential dangers of an untreated or insufficiently treated infection. Especially in cases of HIV and syphilis.

Gonorrhea
Signs and symptoms

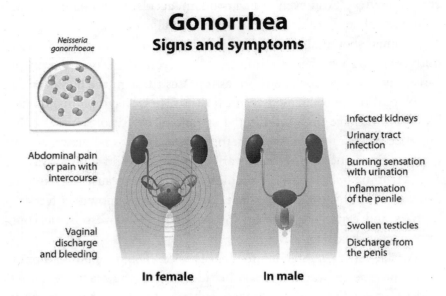

Neisseria gonorrhoeae

Abdominal pain or pain with intercourse

Vaginal discharge and bleeding

In female

Infected kidneys

Urinary tract infection

Burning sensation with urination

Inflammation of the penile

Swollen testicles

Discharge from the penis

In male

Gonorrhea is usually easy to identify due to the pustular discharge and severe painful urination that accompanies it.

TREATMENT OF GENITOURINARY TRACT INFECTIONS

GENERAL MEASURES FOR TREATING UTIS

Let's start with the treatment of urinary tract infections. UTIs are the most common infection in the United States. So, the odds of you getting one, especially if you are female, are really great.

The first thing you need to do is to hydrate yourself, flooding your body with water. This will help to flush out your urinary tract from above, starting with the kidneys, pushing fluid through the ureters, then the bladder, and finally out through the urethra. This will go a long way to mechanically flushing out the pathogens involved.

Eight glasses of water a day is the usual recommendation, but drink as much as you reasonably can, especially during the day. You may want to taper off somewhat at nighttime so you are not up all night, urinating.

If you still feel like you are not urinating enough, add a diuretic like caffeine.

Caffeine, as you know, is found in coffee or black or green tea (herbal teas do not contain caffeine), as well as colas and chocolate. A diuretic is something that increases your urine output, and as everyone knows, coffee and tea certainly fit that description.

Do not hold your urine in; frequent urination will also mechanically flush out your bladder, making it more difficult for bad bacteria to attach to the bladder wall. Drinking unsweetened cranberry juice will also do the same thing.

Cranberry in pill form, known as cranberry extract, can also be used. It comes in 500 mg capsules. Take one capsule twice a day. Cranberry juice has several ingredients such as polyphenols that prevent bacteria from attaching themselves to healthy cells. Drink at least one or two eight-ounce glasses a day.

A little splash of vodka might make it more palatable. Hey, why not have a little fun—life is too damn short. Sometimes, you just have to lighten up and make the best of your situation.

Boosting your immune stimulants such as vitamin C will definitely help a UTI. Vitamin C will acidify your urine, making it a less appealing environment for pathogenic bacteria such as E. coli, which is one of the most frequent invaders.

In addition to which, it will boost your immune system, helping it fight off the infection. Vitamin C also can combine with any nitrates that are present in your urine, forming nitric oxides that rapidly kill bacteria. Don't listen to "the experts" who routinely recommend 100 mg of vitamin C or similar doses. That is plain stupid.

You need to flood your body with vitamin C, which is water soluble, meaning it dissolves in water. And where does that go? Correct, grasshopper, it goes to your kidneys where the excess is urinated out directly into your urinary tract. If you are not on vitamin C already, take 1,000 mg bid (twice a day), I seriously doubt you will get diarrhea from such a dose, but if you do, lower it to 500 mg twice daily. This will ensure your urinary tract is well acidified and flooded with vitamin C, in addition to which, it will stimulate your immune cells to greater bacterial killing.

IODINE, MY NUMBER ONE RECOMMENDATION FOR THE TREATMENT OF UTIS

Another wonderful and very effective way of treating UTIs involves one of my very favorite microbial killers, iodine. A study out of Japan in 2003 indicated the use of various iodine preparations to protect the thyroid in the event of a nuclear explosion.

What I found fascinating was their mention of the urinary excretion of iodine. They found that potassium iodide tablets had a much greater urinary excretion than iodine-rich foods such as kelp. If we can get our kidneys to excrete iodine into our urine, it will kill everything in the urinary tract, including bacteria, fungi, and viruses.

Nothing survives the onslaught of iodine, that is why it is still used to this day for the sterilization of surfaces and as a preop skin prep. Every cell in our bodies utilizes iodine, highlighting its importance to our health.

What I strongly recommend for the treatment of UTIs is using potassium iodide tablets, which are readily available without a prescription. They studied both potassium iodide solution (Lugol's solution) or tablets known as Iodoral. Iodoral or potassium iodide tablets typically come in 12.5 mg doses, but 50 mg high-potency doses are also available.

You can even use nascent iodine drops in water. It is much harder to dose the Lugol's and the nascent. Each drop of Lugol's solution contains a total of 2.5 mg of iodine in its various forms. Each drop of nascent iodine contains 0.4 mg of iodine. So, you would need five drops of Lugol's to be the equivalent of one 12.5 mg Iodoral tablet.

For nascent iodine, you would need thirty-one drops to be the equivalent of a 12.5 mg Iodoral tablet. Naturally, this is to be mixed in water, as much or as little as you like. I think an eight-ounce glass size would be ideal, but to each his own. It simply changes the amount it is diluted in, not the dose.

For a UTI, I would suggest to take one 12.5 mg Iodoral tablet twice a day for a week. That will sterilize your urinary tract, killing all pathogens. I don't think you will need 50 mg of Iodoral, but if that is the only size you have, take it once a day for three days then stop it.

In my opinion, this is by far the best treatment for UTIs. It also prevents the development of resistant bacteria. Since iodine is immediately deadly upon contact, there is no opportunity for bacteria to develop resistance. If you are one of those people (the vast majority of whom are women) who suffers from recurrent UTIs, then one Iodoral tablet, or its equivalent in the form of Lugol's solution or nascent iodine once weekly, should do the trick to prevent recurrence.

American physicians typically are fearful of the use of iodine supplements due to possible side effects on the thyroid, either causing hypothyroidism (slow thyroid) or hyperthyroidism (an overactive thyroid). However, the vast majority of physicians and midlevel providers do not test iodine levels even in their patients with known thyroid disease, Hashimoto's thyroiditis, dry eyes, fibrocystic breasts, or patients with cysts in ovaries and other organs, all of which are caused by iodine deficiency.

The vast majority of people worldwide are deficient in iodine, unless their diets are seafood based, like the Japanese. The world's soils are severely depleted, especially those farthest inland from an ocean. Since it is not replaced by farmers, food grown on those soils are severely iodine deficient.

Almost all my patients that I check iodine levels on are depleted. I find iodine supplementation to be very safe, especially at 12.5 mg Iodoral daily dose (or other equivalent form of iodine). The Japanese diet includes large amounts of seafood and seaweed, both of which are large sources of iodine.

The average Japanese woman has an intake of 13.8 mg of iodine daily from dietary sources. That is on average, meaning half of them have higher intakes. They have very low levels of breast cancer, cysts of all types, and thyroid disease and none of the side effects American physicians worry about, so I feel confident in my recommendations, especially in light of the protean benefits of iodine administration.

However, I would not routinely take higher levels of iodine than I have recommended since it may very well interfere with thyroid function.

UVA URSI

Another good treatment for UTIs is the medicinal plant called uvaursi (*Arctostaphylos uva-ursi*) or its common name, bearberry. It has multiple effects: it is antibacterial, also works as an astringent or drying agent, a diuretic, and also an anti-inflammatory agent. It works best in an alkaline environment; hence I would avoid taking vitamin C if you are using this to treat a UTI.

One way around that is to use Ester-C instead of traditional ascorbic acid form of vitamin C. Ester-C is pH neutral and thus nonacidic and will not adversely affect the uvaursi. Ester-C is a good form of vitamin C to use, if you are one of those rare people who gets GI upset from the normal ascorbic acid form of vitamin C.

Uvaursi should be avoided in women who are pregnant or trying to get pregnant or women breastfeeding and also in children.

Uvaursi comes in various preparations; here are the doses:

Tea: steep three grams of uvaursi tea in five ounces of water for approximately twelve hours then strain, and you can drink it either cold or hot, three or four teacups a day for a maximum of five days. Do not take it any longer and do not use a higher dose; it may cause liver damage.

Tincture: take 5 ml of tincture in water four times a day for a maximum duration of five days. The amount of water used is up to you.

Capsules: capsules come with a standardized dose of the active ingredient arbutin. Take the equivalent of 250 mg of arbutin four times a day for five days maximum.

OREGANO OIL AND COCONUT OIL

Another good treatment is oil of oregano, sometimes called origanum oil (from its botanical name *Origanum vulgare*) or oregano oil. Oregano oil is known to have strong antibacterial effects. What is lesser known is its antiviral, antifungal, antiparasitic, and even anti-inflammatory properties. It has been used for centuries to treat UTIs in China and other countries.

In a very interesting study published in 2005 in the *Toxicology Journal*, they studied the effects of oregano oil and also of monolaurin (from coconuts), separately and together, and even compared them to the use of the very strong antibiotic vancomycin. They also compared other essential oils and found that oregano oil was by far the most effective in treating UTIs.

They also found that combining oregano oil with monolaurin was more potent than either one alone. Another study showed oregano oil to be effective in killing twenty different strains of E. coli and *Pseudomonas aeruginosa*, two of the most common causes of UTIs.

Note: Pregnant and nursing mothers should avoid using oregano oil since it could harm the fetus and will dry up breast milk production. It should also be used cautiously in diabetics since it is also known to lower blood glucose levels. If you are using anticoagulants or blood thinners of any type, you should avoid oregano oil since it may prolong bleeding.

For the same reason, avoid using oregano oil for ten days before any surgery. Avoid oregano oil if you happen to be allergic to mint, sage, marjoram, and basil since your allergies may also cross-react with oregano.

Here are the doses of oregano oil and monolaurin. For oregano oil, take 500 mg capsules four times a day until cured. If you are using the oil form, put three drops in a glass of water or any other liquid (to mask its strong taste), take this once daily for a maximum of two weeks.

Monolaurin derived from coconut oil has been shown to have antibacterial, antifungal (especially against *Candida albicans*), and antiviral activity. For the treatment of UTIs of both bacterial and fungal origin, use 600 mg monolaurin capsules; take two capsules three times a day for ten days. Monolaurin is best absorbed when taken with food.

A NOTE ON THE HERXHEIMER REACTION

Any rapid sudden mass killing/die-off of any bacteria, fungus, or virus has the potential to trigger what is known as a Herxheimer reaction. This is caused by the destruction of these microorganisms and consequently the release of their endotoxins and lipids faster than they can be eliminated by the kidneys or detoxified by the liver.

The symptoms are flulike, with body aches, extreme fatigue, and headaches. The good news is that this means you have just kicked the ass of whatever bug was infecting you. The even better news is that it only lasts a few days and is not harmful to you in any way.

TREATMENT OF HERPES INFECTIONS

The key vulnerability of herpes viruses is their need for the amino acid arginine, as I mentioned earlier in this chapter. Arginine is essential for the herpes virus to reproduce. Without it, its replication is impossible. L-lysine blocks the uptake of arginine.

Hence other than antiviral medications such as acyclovir (brand name Zovirax) and valacyclovir (brand name Valtrex), it is our best shot at forcing a herpes infection into remission. I would take 500 mg of L-lysine three times a day along with the same dose of vitamin C. After three days, double the vitamin C. Remember, it too has antiviral properties.

In addition to which, I would suggest to start zinc and quercetin as soon as possible for its wonderful antiviral effects. Followed by the rest of the gang of seven. By the way, this will also work against any herpes virus family members such as chickenpox and herpes zoster, better known as shingles.

Note: Topical antiviral creams, in my experience, are worthless against a herpes outbreak, other than for soothing the skin. If your skin is raw, you are better off using the closest to pure aloe vera gel you can get and apply that up to three times a day.

I like to keep it in the refrigerator since cold aloe vera feels even better. It does nothing as far as treating the herpes virus but will help heal damaged skin. Zinc 25 mg day and mixed collagen powder 5 grams a day along with at least one gram (1,000 mg) of vitamin C two or three times a day will also help your skin heal from any damage.

Remember, if you use any oral zinc for more than a few weeks, you have to add supplemental copper at about 1 mg daily. The reason being that zinc antagonizes the uptake of copper, which your body needs.

TREATMENT OF VENEREAL DISEASES

Since venereal diseases comprise a wide variety of different pathogens—some being viral, others being bacterial and some even protozoal—that changes our approach, depending upon which one you are infected with. I would also remind you that you and your partner both need to be treated, or you will obviously reinfect one another.

NOTE: If you think you have a venereal disease of any type, I would strongly advise you to seek treatment from a physician or midlevel provider such as a physician's assistant or a nurse practitioner. The reason being that you should be tested to see what you really are infected with in order to more appropriately direct your treatment.

You should also be tested for HIV to rule that out. Infection with two or more venereal diseases at the same time is a common finding.

Examples of bacterial venereal diseases include gonorrhea, chlamydia, campylobacter, shigella, chancroid, granuloma inguinale and syphilis. Some such as syphilis are extremely dangerous if inadequately treated and may result in damage to multiple organs including the brain, liver, eyes, nervous system, bones, joints, and blood vessels.

Syphilis is known as the great imitator since it has so many different manifestations and symptoms. It also goes through various stages where someone might think they are cured.

All the abovenamed bacterial venereal diseases will need antibiotics to be treated appropriately, such as penicillin, erythromycin, azithromycin, cephalosporins, and doxycycline. Adequate treatment of these venereal infections unfortunately is beyond the scope of this book.

However, if you are in a situation where you cannot get to a physician's office, clinic, or hospital and need to treat it in the meantime, then I would suggest following all the earlier recommendations I made for treating a UTI, especially the use of high-dose iodine. I would advise to use 25 mg (two of the 12.5 mg tablets) of Iodoral or its equivalent in Lugol's or nascent iodine drops twice a day for a maximum of seven to ten days.

I would also treat any skin outbreaks with topical iodine (Betadine) and go on the gang of seven immune-boosting superstars to aid your immune system in eradicating this infection.

Remember, these are only stopgap measures to be used until you can get to a doctor and get tested and properly diagnosed and appropriately treated. Do not mess around with this. If it is syphilis or HIV, the consequences are very serious, including death. In addition to which, you do not want to be a vector for these infections, spreading them to your sex partners.

Treatment of viral or parasitic venereal infections requires a different approach. Examples of sexually transmitted viral infections include herpes, hepatitis B, HIV, and human papillomavirus (HPV). I explained the best way to treat herpes infections earlier in this section. HIV and hepatitis will need an immediate evaluation by a physician.

In the interim, I would immediately start the gang of seven and some oral iodine discussed earlier. The use of quercetin and zinc will help treat any viral infection, but it is not a cure. Genital warts are caused by HPV, which currently has seventy different subtypes.

The warts themselves need to be destroyed either by freezing them off with cryotherapy or burning them off with an electrocautery device such as a Bovie. Either way, you will most likely need to get this treated by a physician.

There are over the counter treatments for warts of all types, including venereal; but in my experience, they do not work very well. Many contain salicylic acid, which is derived from aspirin. They are available over the counter. You have to be very careful not to damage the surrounding healthy skin. Discontinue its use if the surrounding skin gets irritated. You may protect the healthy skin by covering it with a thin film of Vaseline.

The category of sexually transmitted parasitic or protozoal infections includes a single agent trichomonas vaginalis which causes the infection known as trichomoniasis. Trichomoniasis is the most common sexually transmitted disease. The only good news is that it is fairly benign and does not cause many complications.

The most effective treatment for trichomoniasis is a single dose of either metronidazole (trade name Flagyl) or tinidazole (trade name Tindamax) antibiotics. Both are by prescription and will also treat bacterial vaginal infections.

Trichomoniasis can also be treated with iodine. Betadine mixed in water is used as a vaginal douche and is very effective since it is universally deadly to bacteria, fungi, parasites such as the protozoa trichomonas and even viruses. That explains why Betadine or iodine douches are so effective against any kind of vaginal infection and should be your first go-to treatment.

An alternative method is to use a Betadine-soaked tampon. Insert the tampon into your vagina and leave it there for a half an hour, twice a day for a week. Men can also soak a Q-tip in Betadine and gently (ever so gently) insert it just inside the opening of their urethra at the tip of their penis.

Perhaps a better alternative for many of us is to manually stretch open the opening of the urethra and, using a dropper, drip a few drops of Betadine into it. Men can also clean the outside of their penises with a Betadine-soaked cotton ball.

The only possible problem is eradication of the trichomonas from sites outside the vagina, such as the urethra (of both you and your partner) and Bartholin's glands. To eradicate any infection from those sites, I would suggest to take oral iodine as I described earlier for UTIs.

The more prolonged the contact between the Betadine and the microorganisms, the greater the killing capacity. That is the reason for instilling it into your vagina and waiting as long as you can before allowing it to run out. The ideal position is lying on your back and raising your hips, with pillows propped under you to hold you comfortably in position.

Be aware that Betadine will stain clothing, sheets, and towels a dark brown. Doing this in an empty bathtub might reduce the mess. To further enhance the killing power of Betadine, do it two times a day for one to two weeks, depending on your response.

As the Betadine breaks down, it releases free iodine that is toxic to the invading germs, but not to the good vaginal flora such as lactobacilli. Lactobacilli usually recolonize the vagina in as little as two or three hours after treatment with a Betadine douche. They keep the normal pH of the vagina moderately acidic, and they kill bad bacteria and fungi by producing both lactic acid (hence their name) and hydrogen peroxide.

In my lifelong study of the human body and its intricate function, I have noticed that nature repeatedly uses the same useful molecules such as hydrogen peroxide. Thus I think it behooves us to mimic nature as much as possible in our search for effective treatments.

How to make a Betadine vaginal douche: There are several ways to make your Betadine vaginal douche; the easiest way is to buy the premixed brand-name Betadine vaginal douche. It comes with the applicator bottle and instructions. You are essentially mixing 30 cc (or ml) of Betadine with 250 cc of warm water.

You insert the applicator into your vagina and squeeze the air out of the bottle holding your mixture. Then gently remove the applicator tip from your vagina and allow the bottle to refill itself with air; reinsert the applicator and repeat the process. Do this until the bottle is empty. Note that 250 cc is slightly more than a cup. If you are mixing it yourself, just use a 10 percent mix—that is nine parts water to one part Betadine.

Remember, you can use iodine in a number of places, even your mouth and throat. If you have vaginal or penile symptoms of a venereal infection and have also engaged in oral sex with that same partner, then there is a good chance you have also an infection in your mouth and throat.

For that problem, you can turn to our old friend iodine once again and make a solution to gargle with. As I mentioned earlier in chapter 6, there is a premade product for this known as Betadine Sore Throat Gargle, or you can simply mix a 10 percent solution of Betadine and water. As you recall, that is one part Betadine to nine parts water. Pour the mix into your mouth and tilt your head back and gargle it and make sure to swish it around your tongue and all your teeth and hold it for thirty seconds. Do this twice a day for seven to ten days.

CHAPTER TEN

GASTROINTESTINAL INFECTIONS

Gastrointestinal or GI infections technically include everything from the mouth to the anus. However, under respiratory tract infections, we have already covered how to treat mouth and throat infections. Hence in this chapter, we will learn how to treat infections of the stomach, small and large intestines, and finally the rectum and anus.

I always like to acquaint my readers with the anatomy of the area we are considering, so let's take a look at the anatomy of the GI tract.

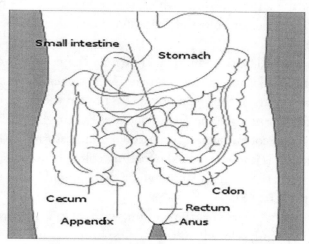

The anatomy of the GI tract, courtesy of *Wikipedia*.

Let's follow some food through the GI tract from its entry point in the mouth to its exit from the anus:

Food enters the mouth and is chewed and transferred to the back of the mouth (upper throat), which is called the oral pharynx. This food is chewed up well and mixed with saliva that has enzymes that begin to digest the starches in the food.

The food then proceeds down the esophagus to the stomach. In the stomach, it is partially decomposed and digested by strong acids. It leaves the stomach and enters the first part of the small intestine. The small intestine has three parts: the first is the duodenum, the second is the jejunum, and the final is the ileum.

If the food contains fat, a signal is sent to the gallbladder, causing it to contract, squirting out bile to digest the fat. In this part of the small intestine, the food will be further digested by enzymes from the pancreas. There are three types of pancreatic digestive enzymes: those that will digest fats (lipases), proteins (proteases), and starches (amylases).

In the small intestine, the pH is the opposite of the acidic stomach; it is a high pH or alkaline area. As food exits the ileum, it enters the first part of the large intestine, which is also known as the colon. The colons job is to reabsorb most of the water mixed in with the food and some minerals.

The first small part is an area known as the cecum, from which extends a fingerlike protrusion known as the appendix. As the food enters the next part of the colon, it goes up toward the head, and this is known as the ascending colon. Then it crosses from right to left, and this is the transverse colon. It then turns down and heads toward the anus, and this section is known as the descending colon, from which it enters an S-shaped section, which is known as the sigmoid colon (*sigmoid* is Greek for the letter *S*).

Then the final section is the rectum, with its lower doorway being the anus, hopefully closed by the anal sphincter until it senses the pressure of feces building up, at which time it will dilate and open, allowing a bowel movement to occur.

Food is propelled along the GI tract by a wave of successive contractions and relaxations of each section. This is known as peristalsis.

When the GI tract is irritated, it often leads to a speeding up of peristalsis with an outpouring of fluid, causing diarrhea. Stimulants like caffeine can also speed up peristalsis.

The opposite effect or a slowing down of peristalsis or a complete shutdown of peristalsis known as ileus can be caused by opiates. Ileus often accompanies GI surgeries. Ileus causes the shutdown of peristalsis and results in absolutely no bowel movements or even flatus (gas) being passed. It also reverses the direction of peristalsis, causing vomiting. The good news is that it only lasts one to three days; the bad news is that when it is happening to you, you are so miserable, it seems like it lasts forever!

Peristalsis is also helped along by the contents of the stool. A healthy stool should have a large quantity of fiber in it; this draws in water and keeps the stool wet and also gives it structure. A healthy stool should be medium -brown in color and floats in the toilet. If it sinks, it does not have enough fiber content. Fiber is also incredibly useful as a prebiotic or a food to feed your good intestinal bacteria or your intestinal flora.

Fiber is not digested by our body and thus remains intact in healthy stool. The optimal amount of fiber in your diet should be approximately 30 to 40 grams a day. Most Americans get less than half of that. To get more, increase the fruits, whole grains, and vegetables in your diet.

Raw vegetables and fruit are better than processed since they also contain enzymes that are essential to helping you properly digest food. A dry, hard stool is difficult to pass, but a moist soft stool travels through your GI tract with ease. That is why a diet containing a large amount of fruit and vegetables and adequate water is the best cure for constipation.

No amount of fiber will work to cure constipation if it does not have enough water to draw in to make it soft. If you take fiber supplements without drinking enough water, it will form a plug that will severely constipate you and may even obstruct your bowels.

Some general considerations to keep in mind when you want to better understand the GI tract, as odd as it sounds: it is a hollow tube running from your mouth to your anus. Nutrients such as carbohydrates, fats, and protein, along with minerals and water, are absorbed from your food.

In order to be absorbed, nutrients must cross a single layer of cells known as enterocytes that line our intestines. The body has specific ways to allow what it needs to be absorbed, rejecting the rest. What's absorbed is the only part that is actually entering your body. Anything passed along, like fiber, goes through without ever getting inside.

Isn't that so weird? Illustrating that point, I once read about an Australian in 1970 named Leon Sampson. He was a circus strongman, and he bet another fellow $20,000 that he could eat an entire Volkswagen! It took him four years to collect, but he ate it all—tires, glass, interior, even the radio. He did it by grinding it into very minute sand-like grains and mixing it with his soup or mashed potatoes. It didn't hurt him because it never was absorbed into his body but rather passed through it. YOUR GI TRACT IS ALL ABOUT ABSORPTION. Sorry for screaming, trying to emphasize that point and driving it home to you!

That is why chewing your food and eating slowly is so important. It grinds the food into small-enough pieces. Small pieces allow digestive enzymes a greater surface area to make contact with the food and further break it down into absorbable portions the body can handle.

You can also get enzymes that will aid in your digestion from raw fruit and vegetables. What a great design! Food that nurtures us also provides a better way for it to be digested by packing its nutrients with enzymes. Those same enzymes are destroyed at temperatures around 130 degrees F, even for a short period.

My lovely wife, Lynne, makes some outrageous salads, mixing raw vegetables, fruit, nuts, and seeds. With a delicious dressing, it tastes great, and is healthy to boot.

The fiber in raw vegetables also acts as a prebiotic, or a food for your probiotic bacteria. Prebiotics such as fiber are not digested and pass intact into the intestines, essentially feeding the bacteria living there. These good bacteria are ingenious little bastards. They take the prebiotic and ferment it, releasing previously unavailable nutrients that they require to thrive!

Some foods that are excellent prebiotics include asparagus, bananas, chicory root, dandelions, fennel, garlic, most beans, nuts, Jerusalem artichokes (affectionately called fartichokes for obvious reasons), sauerkraut, and all members of the onion family such as onions, leeks, shallots, and scallions.

Yogurt with live cultures and fermented foods are full of good prebiotic food as well as lots of probiotic bacteria. Dark chocolate is also a good prebiotic food. Now that got your attention, didn't it? Next chance you get, I can hear you already. "Honey, pass me that dark chocolate. Did you know it is a health food?"

Probiotics are the good bacteria that line our gut and predigests food that is passing through, taking what it needs and giving the rest to you. They also produce B vitamins, especially B12 and other vitamins such as K2 that are essential for our health.

Since they line the intestines, they occupy this territory as their own, preventing colonization and infections by other pathogens. That is a huge help to our immune system. That is why antibiotics are so bad for us—they indiscriminately kill off most bacteria, both good and bad.

Once your intestinal flora (the good bacteria and even some fungi that live in our gut) is damaged or eradicated in areas, it results in pioneer bacteria and fungi invading and colonizing the gut lining, thus damaging its function as a protective barrier.

One of the most important functions of your microbiome is to keep the single layer of epithelial cells lining our intestines in good health. When those cells are damaged, it results in large undigested portions of proteins being absorbed right into the blood.

This is called leaky gut syndrome, and it is the most likely cause of the skyrocketing numbers of people with allergies, asthma, and autoimmune diseases of all kinds. What happens is those large undigested pieces of protein trigger an antibody attack and subsequent activation of the immune system.

For example, if a segment of protein is similar to a protein on the surface of a thyroid cell, it causes antithyroid antibodies to be produced, which then attack the thyroid injuring it, leading to inflammation and ultimately Hashimoto's thyroiditis.

I could write an entire book just about the benefits and wonders of our intestinal microbiome, but alas, I won't. Suffice it to say that keeping your gut microflora in tip-top condition will prevent obesity; prevent disease; prevent asthma, allergies, autoimmune diseases; promote health;

and increase your absorption of life-giving nutrients. A pretty good deal for both us and them—what is known as a symbiotic relationship, one in which both parties benefit.

SYMPTOMS OF GASTROINTESTINAL INFECTIONS

STOMACH INFECTION

The primary infection of the stomach is from the bacteria *Helicobacter pylori*. When I was first out of medical school, the dogma at the time was that germs could not survive the strong acid of the stomach. Ulcers of the stomach and duodenum were thought to be due to excess acid, stress, alcohol, and a poor diet.

Two Australian doctors made the discovery that indeed it was this bacterium that caused peptic ulcers and not lifestyle. It was such a revelation that it won them the Nobel Prize for Medicine in 2005.

The overwhelming majority (greater than 90 percent) of patients have no idea that they are infected with *Helicobacter pylori*. How it is spread is remains an enigma. The assumption is that it is spread via oral-oral contact or fecal-oral, but I have had many married couples in my practice where one is infected but not the other. Truth is, we know it is in the saliva and feces, and also in dental plaque, but we have no idea how you actually catch it.

The usual symptoms of an *H. pylori* infection in those who are symptomatic is reflux (heartburn), bloating, abdominal pain, and nausea. In severe cases, it can cause bleeding from the stomach. When blood is exposed to stomach acid, it will turn a black tarry color, which subsequently you will see in your stools.

Bleeding from further down in the intestines and/or anally from hemorrhoids, for example, is easily distinguished by its bright-red color.

H. pylori can be diagnosed easily by either a breath test or blood test of the gold standard, which is a biopsy of the stomach via an upper endoscopy (putting an endoscope down your throat into your stomach).

Left untreated, an *H. pylori* infection can lead to gastric ulcers and, in some patients, stomach cancer and less commonly lymphomas.

GASTROENTERITIS: INFECTIONS OF THE STOMACH AND INTESTINES

There are primarily three types of organisms that infect our gastrointestinal tracts: viral, bacterial, and parasitic. All cause similar symptoms.

One of the most common GI infections is gastroenteritis or what is commonly known as the stomach flu. It has nothing to do with seasonal flu, which is a respiratory tract infection caused by different influenza viruses. Viral gastroenteritis usually causes watery, non-bloody diarrhea, often accompanied by painful abdominal cramps, nausea, and vomiting. Occasionally, it causes a fever, but not very often.

Gastroenteritis is usually something that lasts a day or two, so many folks call it the twenty-four-hour or forty-eight-hour bug or stomach flu. As you can tell by the name, it is short-lived and usually more of an annoyance than a serious problem. However, in infants and the elderly, it can be deadly.

Infants get dehydrated quickly and can easily die, which is often the case in third world countries. The elderly often fall victim to otherwise run-of-the-mill infections like gastroenteritis and seasonal flu infections due to their multiple comorbidities and overall debilitated condition.

The severe diarrhea you find in a gastroenteritis is unfortunately also the hallmark of a host of other bacterial infections including Clostridia difficile, salmonella, shigella, campylobacter, and even parasitic infections like giardiasis.

My point is that without access to a diagnostic laboratory to do stool studies, it is incredibly difficult to tell one cause of diarrhea from another. What they all have in common is that they have waged war on your normal gut flora and won!

When your GI tract is infected, it has a limited number of defense mechanisms it can employ. Its favorite is expelling the offending agent out of the body, either by violent retching and vomiting or explosive diarrhea.

Alternatively, the gut wall can pour out fluid that hopefully will mechanically wash away all or most of the invading bacteria. Both can lead to painful abdominal cramps. Depending upon the infectious agent, sometimes there is bleeding, most frequently in the stool, less frequently in the contents of your vomit.

Occasionally, your body will decide to turn up its furnace and spike a fever, which will hopefully kill off the bacteria or viruses involved since they all live in a very narrow temperature range. That is why I have repeatedly said never to treat a fever but rather let it burn; it is one of your body's greatest defense mechanism to eradicate an infectious agent of any type.

FOODBORNE ILLNESSES OR FOOD POISONING

Foodborne illnesses are caused from a variety of factors. It can involve bacteria, viruses, parasites, spoiled food, undercooked foods such as beans, and toxins in foods from improper canning or contamination. One major source worldwide is from the ingestion of poisonous mushrooms from misidentification. Many mushrooms are very similar in appearances, and novices often mistake one variety for another. This can be a deadly mistake.

Food poisoning is not rare, and patients often present with it in my office. What is rare is the patient who is able to identify the source, which usually happens only when the entire family becomes sick after eating the same meal.

Most people attribute their symptoms to their last meal. That is usually not the case due to the incubation period for the various pathogens (germs) that cause food poisoning. Among them, the shortest incubation period is approximately eight hours for *Clostridium perfringens* and the longest being up to seven days for campylobacter. Hence the problem with identifying its source.

DIVERTICULOSIS AND ITS EVIL COUSIN DIVERTICULITIS

Diverticulosis is a condition that produces saclike projections (diverticula) outward from the wall of the colon. It is thought to be caused by a low-fiber diet that produces increased intraluminal pressure (inside the gut), pushing out against the wall.

They often form where blood vessels penetrate the muscular wall of the colon, creating an area of structural weakness. The combination of a low-fiber diet and structural weakness create the perfect storm for a blowout of the wall, leading to the creation of these marble-sized pouches.

The same poor diet also changes the bacteria in the gut, leading to inflammation of the gut wall, weakening it, and also predisposing you to diverticulosis. Diverticulosis is almost nonexistent in the third world and was nonexistent in the Western world up until modern times.

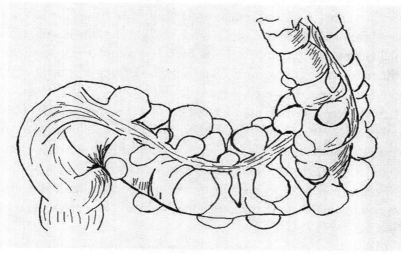

Drawing showing multiple diverticular sacs of the
sigmoid colon compliments of *Wikipedia*.

Diverticulosis is the condition of multiple diverticula primarily in the colon. When these diverticula become chronically inflamed or acutely infected, it is known as diverticulitis. Diverticulosis is asymptomatic, meaning it has no symptoms.

About 10 to 25 percent of patients with diverticulosis go on at some point to develop diverticulitis. The cause of diverticulitis is unknown. Previously, it was felt to be secondary to eating hard nuts, seeds, or popcorn; currently, that is felt not to be the case. However, I disagree.

I cannot tell you how many times I see patients with diverticulitis who develop it several days after eating one of those three. Mechanically, it makes sense since the nuts, seeds, or popcorn get stuck in the opening of the diverticulum, sealing it off. After which, the contents of the pouch fester and an infection develops.

Symptoms of diverticulitis almost always involve abdominal pain, most frequently on the left lower quadrant of the abdomen/pelvis. Many times, it is severe enough to prompt a visit to the emergency room. That being said, the threshold for going to the ER varies wildly from patient to patient. Some go to the ER for the most minor problems; others, not until they are almost terminal.

The reason for the left-sided location is the greater intraluminal pressure on the left, hence the greater frequency of left-side diverticula over the right. The intraluminal pressure is greatest on the left due to several factors. Primary of which is a law of physics, the law of Laplace, which states that the pressure in a tube is greatest where its diameter is the narrowest. The sigmoid located in the left lower quadrant of the abdomen is the narrowest point of the colon.

A Western diet high in processed foods and refined carbohydrates is consequently very low in fiber. Without the presence of undigested fiber to pull in water, the stools are hard and are difficult to move through the gut. To propel them along, the large muscles of the colon wall have to strongly contract, once again increasing the intraluminal pressure. The combination of all these factors produces the preponderance of left-sided diverticula.

Other less frequent symptoms are fever, nausea, vomiting, and sometimes some bleeding. It is not a rare condition, and I see it very frequently in my clinical practice. Many of my patients have recurrent bouts of diverticulitis. Despite what the "experts" say, I tell them to limit their intake of hard nuts, seeds, and popcorn as well as increasing their fluid and fiber and in many cases. It almost completely eliminates future recurrences.

INFECTIONS OF THE RECTUM AND ANUS

There are several types of infections of the rectum, anus, and perianal (around the anus) areas. I am not including here venereal infections of all types, which is beyond the scope of this book and almost always a consequence of anal sex. Common sexually transmitted infections in this area include herpes virus infections, syphilis, gonorrhea, chlamydia, and HIV.

If you are a homosexual or a heterosexual who has anal intercourse, you are essentially introducing a penis into an area of the body that is not designed to accommodate one. This has consequences, including structural damage to the anal sphincter, tearing of the anus or rectum, and the introduction of venereal diseases of every variety.

If you are engaging in this type of sexual activity and you develop an infection of some type, then you should consult either your primary care provider or your gynecologist.

Oftentimes, anal sex can lead to inflammation and infection of the rectum known as proctitis. The symptoms are painful bowel movements, and depending upon the infectious agent, it can cause mucus and or pustular discharge and, less often, bleeding.

Patients oftentimes feel like they need to have frequent bowel movements and very little or nothing comes out. Proctitis is predominantly caused by anal sex, but sometimes the cause is not sexual as in the case of dysentery, which is caused by infection with an amoeba.

Infections can still develop in patients who are not engaging in anally receptive sex. That is the purpose of this section.

By far, in a primary care setting like my office, the most common infections of the anus and the perianal area are fungal in origin. Patients will experience intense itching of the anus and surrounding skin, oftentimes with some redness and mild soft tissue swelling indicating the involved areas.

Intense scratching may open up the skin and allow bacteria to invade, leading to a bacterial infection of the skin or what is known as a cellulitis, but that is not as common. These bacterial infections can lead to deeper collections of pus or abscesses in the perianal area. An abscess in this area will appear as an olive-sized swelling that is very tender and even painful to touch, similar to a skin boil.

Painful swelling inside your anus and tissue adjacent to it and just outside of it are most often caused by hemorrhoids. Hemorrhoids are essentially veins in your anus and outside of it whose walls lack muscle and often will stretch out and become enlarged and swollen. There are two types of hemorrhoids: external and internal.

External hemorrhoids can be felt when you are washing or wiping yourself—they feel like swollen, oftentimes painful areas around the outside of your anus. External hemorrhoids often bleed, and bright-red blood is often noted on the toilet paper or inside the toilet bowl. Both types of hemorrhoids can be itchy at times.

External hemorrhoids often develop clots inside of them. This is known as thrombosis. That is more of a problem, and if real severe, i.e., very large and painful—they may require surgical correction. Thrombosis more often occurs in external hemorrhoids but can also occur in internal hemorrhoids and is a common presenting problem in primary care offices.

If the thrombosis is partial, it can be treated; but if completely involving the entire hemorrhoid, this is a complete thrombosis and oftentimes requires surgical banding or actual surgery.

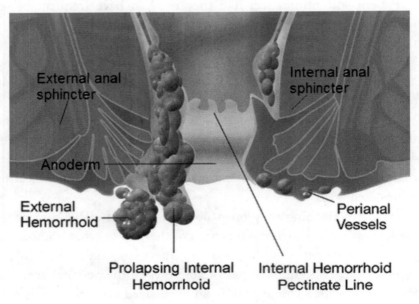

Drawing compliments of *Wikipedia*.

Internal hemorrhoids are located inside the anus, and to be felt, one has to insert a finger (hopefully gloved) an inch or so inside the anus. Internal hemorrhoids oftentimes bleed, always a bright-red color blood, usually noted by patients on their toilet paper. They, oftentimes, are very itchy as well. To add to patients' confusion, they oftentimes get large and flop out of the anus, which is called prolapsing. If an internal hemorrhoid prolapses, it can be felt on the outside.

Hemorrhoids are not caused by infection but most often from straining bowel movements during constipation, sitting on the toilet for prolonged periods, pregnancy, recurrent bouts of either diarrhea or constipation, and anal sex. A poor diet low in fiber can cause constipation and, in turn, lead to hemorrhoids. I have included hemorrhoids in this section of GI infections because it is a commonly occurring pathology that oftentimes confuses patients.

If there is an infection in the lower GI tract area, i.e., the anus and rectum, the most common symptom is itching. Other symptoms are bleeding, pain, redness to the involved area, mucus discharge, pustular discharge, and spasm of the area in and around the anus.

TREATMENT OF GASTROINTESTINAL INFECTIONS

Infections of the upper GI tract such as the stomach such as *Helicobacter pylori* are difficult to properly treat without the use of antibiotics. Eradication of an *H. pylori* infection is important because if left untreated, they may lead to peptic ulcers and even ultimately to stomach cancer.

Infections with *H. pylori* usually require treatment with two antibiotics and Pepto-Bismol four times a day, without which, the antibiotics will not properly work since Pepto-Bismol contains bismuth, which helps eradicate *Helicobacter pylori*.

Two antibiotics are needed due to the rise of antibiotic resistance among *Helicobacter pylori*. *H. pylori* infections are especially prominent in third world countries.

H. pylori infections also require a stomach acid–reducing regimen such as use of proton pump inhibitors (PPIs) such as omeprazole (Prilosec), lansoprazole (Prevacid), esomeprazole (Nexium), rabeprazole (Aciphex), dexlansoprazole (Dexilant), and pantoprazole (Protonix). Also H2 blockers such as Pepcid (famotidine), Tagamet (cimetidine),

Axid (nizatidine), and Zantac (ranitidine) also work to lower stomach acid levels but are not as potent as the PPIs.

Oral antacids such as Tums, Maalox, or Mylanta will also work, but to a much lesser degree and aren't as well tolerated and may lead to diarrhea. All the above treatments will also help reduce symptoms of reflux or heartburn. They also help reduce symptoms of bloating, which frequently accompany gastritis and gastric infections.

Probiotics will also help with all gastrointestinal infections since they help colonize the GI tract and thus compete with pathogenic or disease-causing bacteria for territory, resulting in their inhibition. The most useful of the probiotic bacteria are the lactic acid bacteria such as lactobacillus and bifidobacterium.

If you are using probiotics to treat your GI infections, make sure they ae included. That shouldn't be too difficult since they are the most common. They are completely resistant to the strong acidic environment of the stomach and are naturally occurring in healthy GI tracts.

Furthermore, probiotics work by supporting the mucosal lining of the stomach by their secretion of short-chain fatty acids and other antibacterial substances that inhibit *H. pylori*. Remember, yogurt and fermented foods such as kimchi, kefir, and kombucha all contain significant amounts of beneficial probiotic bacteria along with many other health-promoting substances.

My secret weapon against all GI infections is activated charcoal. It is used universally in emergency rooms to neutralize ingested poisons and to treat overdoses, but has many other uses medicinally.

Activated charcoal works due to its immense surface area on which chemicals and toxins of all types adsorb. Adsorbing means that it bonds almost all chemicals, toxins, and even bacteria on its surface.

Adsorption is different from absorption, which means it takes up the substance and mechanically swells. Activated charcoal does not do that, so it does not cause bloating or other problems. It is incredibly potent and will work even with alcohol to bind and detoxify it.

Take two capsules before you go out drinking for the evening, and you will immediately note that you have not caught a buzz at all since it is adsorbed and does not enter your bloodstream.

The one caveat to remember when taking activated charcoal is the two-hour rule. You cannot use it within two hours of taking a medication since it will neutralize it. That means if you take it now, any meds you took up to two hours ago may be neutralized, and you cannot take any other meds for two hours after you use it for the same reason.

Activated charcoal works almost immediately to help symptoms of nausea and vomiting. I have utilized it for decades in my office. Patients come in sick as hell, and to their utter amazement, within a short time, they are back to normal. It will also help with diarrhea, but not with constipation. It is very effective against food poisoning of all types, neutralizing the toxins produced by the pathogenic bacteria.

Another treatment for nausea, which usually accompanies upper GI infections more than lower, is marijuana. Pot has been used for years for cancer patients to help alleviate the nausea and vomiting accompanying chemotherapy. It is quite effective and, as of late, has been legalized in many states and decriminalized in many others. Think back, were you ever nauseous during the seventies? Now you know why!

Nausea is also helped by oral antacids such as Mylanta, Maalox, and Tums. One of my favorites is the spice ginger, such as in ginger ale. It can also be eaten raw, comes in tablets, or you can use ground ginger. The dose of which is one quarter to one-half of a teaspoon as often as you need it. Usually every four to six hours. It will also help alleviate inflammation, motion sickness, and intestinal spasms.

Baking soda or sodium bicarbonate can also be used to treat nausea and gastric upset. Baking soda is very alkaline (the opposite of acidic) and, as such, will help neutralize stomach acids. It is thus especially useful in gastritis (stomach inflammation) as well as gastric infections and peptic ulcers.

I would suggest starting very low with a quarter of a teaspoon in an eight-ounce glass of water; increase it to a max of half a teaspoon. You can take this four to six times a day; however (this is very important), do not take it if your stomach is distended (enlarged) and bloated since it produces gas and may actually lead to violent vomiting and possibly even stomach rupture.

You can even concoct your own effervescent antacid by using the following recipe taken from an excellent book called *Baking Soda: Over*

500 Fabulous, Fun, and Frugal Uses You've Probably Never Thought Of by Victor Lansky.

Take an 8 oz glass; add to it the following: one tablespoon of vinegar, one-half teaspoon of sugar, one-half teaspoon of baking soda, and one-half cup of water. Drink it immediately after mixing while it is still fizzing.

Once the vomiting is under control, you can soothe your stomach by using chicken soup or broth, apple juice (do not substitute other juices such as orange or grapefruit since they are too acidic). Small amounts of Jell-O also work wonders for soothing your stomach while at the same time providing collagen for your body.

Jell-O is a short-term fix for your collagen needs and contains artificial sweeteners such as aspartame, food dyes, and other chemicals. Gelatin, on the other hand, is collagen that has been heated and structurally changed and is an excellent source of protein, especially collagen.

Gelatin is also available flavored but usually has very little taste to it anyway. Let's face it, you are going to have to go with regular Jell-O or flavored gelatins to get your kids to eat it.

Many patients benefit from using the BRAT diet after a bout of gastritis. BRAT stands for bananas, rice, applesauce, and toast. These foods are easily digested and all are low in fat, protein, and fiber. The bananas are also high in potassium, which is lost in large quantities with any nausea, vomiting, or diarrhea.

Naturally, you should avoid alcohol and NSAIDS (ibuprofen, Motrin, naprosyn, Alleve, Advil, and aspirin), spicy foods, and caffeine, which all can cause GI distress, especially in the stomach. Acetaminophen or Tylenol is okay to use since it does not cause any GI upset.

Milk should also be avoided for at least two days. Despite popular opinion, milk does not help an upset stomach. The milk-digesting enzyme lactase is produced in the stomach lining and gets depleted by gastritis and nausea and vomiting. For this reason, most people suffer from a temporary lactose intolerance following a GI infection. This lasts for about two weeks.

For that reason, dairy products should be avoided to prevent diarrhea for two weeks after a GI infection.

Once you are feeling better, I would suggest to eat lightly for a week—no large meals and no really heavy meals of meat and fat, which will lead to distention of your stomach and possibly a reactivation of your nausea and vomiting.

Gastrointestinal tract infections will invariably lead to a certain degree of dehydration. Either from vomiting or diarrhea, from either end, you are losing large amounts of fluids. Avoid alcohol and caffeine, which will worsen your dehydration, especially caffeine since it is a diuretic (makes you urinate). More fluid loss is the last thing you need.

Your lost fluids need to be replaced before you will feel truly recovered. Hydration is an often overlooked but essential treatment for all GI infections. For hydration, water is fine by itself, but you will benefit even greater from some electrolyte replacement since GI infections lead to diarrhea and vomiting, which deplete chloride, potassium, and sodium in large quantities.

Replacement of sodium, chloride, and potassium is an essential component of your rehydration strategy. Gatorade is fine, in a pinch, but it is not much more than a very high amount of sugar with some sodium and potassium. Probably the best natural rehydration fluid is coconut water.

Coconut water has the same electrolyte consistency as blood plasma. That is very important since we want to rehydrate our body via our blood. Dehydration contracts the water component of our blood and, when caused by GI fluid losses, results in major electrolyte losses.

We want to replace those lost blood electrolytes. Since coconut water contains them, it is a perfect choice. Coconut water is high in both potassium and also in iron. It is also low in sugar (unlike Gatorade). Coconut water is also high in other electrolytes, enzymes, vitamins, minerals, and phytonutrients.

Phyto means coming from a plant source. In addition to approximately three grams of fiber per cup, coconut water is an excellent source of vitamin C. The best coconut water is produced by young coconuts of about five to seven months of age.

Do not confuse coconut water with coconut milk. Coconut milk is made by mixing coconut water with chopped up coconut meat and then squeezing the mixture under pressure. Coconut milk is also a healthy drink, but not our ideal choice for hydration. It is full of minerals, vitamins, and medium-chain triglycerides.

Medium-chain triglycerides are a type of fatty acid that is readily and easily utilized by our bodies. As such, it is an excellent source of fat, which I have emphasized to you many times as being essential for your health.

You can formulate your own rehydration fluid mixes. Here are three examples that you can easily make at home from a few handy items:

Take a liter of water. (A quart is close enough for those of you who are metrically challenged! You see, you should have paid more attention in school.) Add six teaspoons of sugar, one teaspoon of table salt (sodium chloride). One-half teaspoon of salt substitute (potassium chloride). And finally, a quarter teaspoon of baking soda or sodium bicarbonate.

A simpler concoction can also be used. Take one pint of water and add a pinch of salt, a teaspoon of either lemon or lime juice, and finally a teaspoon of sugar. Naturally, to make a quart or liter, just double the above ingredients since there are two pints in a quart.

A third, very simple formula is as follows: Take one quart of water, add one-half teaspoon of table salt, approximately 2.5 grams, then add six teaspoons of sugar, which is approximately 30 grams.

Diarrhea can also be treated with bovine colostrum. Colostrum is the first substance made by the breasts of both humans and cows (bovine). It is followed by normal breast milk in the case of humans and cow's milk in the case of cows. Both types of colostrum are loaded with antibodies from the mother to help protect baby infants and calves from infections of all types.

Bovine colostrum has been found to contain large numbers of antibodies to bacterial, viral, and protozoal pathogens that cause diarrhea. Bovine colostrum will also help heal leaky gut syndrome and thus, in turn, will help those suffering from the many food allergies that usually accompany it.

Iodine, our old friend, once again comes in quite handy to treat infectious diarrhea. Iodine is extremely efficient at killing pathogens of all types and is especially effective against the "bugs" that cause diarrhea. Iodine as a diarrhea treatment is effective in its various forms, including nascent or elemental iodine, Lugol's solution, and even potassium iodide tablets and kelp capsules.

Using nascent iodine solution, you add six to eight drops in a small glass of water and drink this up to four times a day for up to a week. If the diarrhea abates earlier, you can stop it sooner. If you use Lugol's solution, it comes in two strengths: 5 and 2 percent.

Mix six drops of the 5 percent or fifteen drops of the 2 percent in a glass of water; drink this four times a day. For children, cut the above doses in half (iodine is not to be given to infants). The best way to use it is to first swish it around your mouth and then swallow it; this way, it will also disinfect your mouth. It has a slight medicinal taste—get over it, it works well, stop being a wimp.

You should be aware that proper absorption of iodine requires the presence of vitamin C. You should be taking vitamin C already. Hopefully, you are on a gram (1,000 mg) or two of vitamin C. If you are not, then shame on you. Start gradually. I would recommend 500 mg twice a day and work up to the 2,000 mg a day (in two divided doses). Remember, high-dose vitamin C has only one side effect, diarrhea, so make sure you are not making it worse.

Colloidal silver is another way to treat GI infections of all types. Colloidal silver is a mineral drink composed of very small silver particles suspended in a colloid. A colloid is a liquid where all the atoms are equally spaced apart due to their electric charge. Due to the force of those small electric charges, the silver never comes out of solution and settles. Think Jell-O or milk. The material the silver is suspended is the colloid.

Silver has been well known for centuries for its antimicrobial properties, meaning it kills bacteria, viruses, and fungi. Up until the advent of antibiotic era, which began during WWII, silver preparations were widely used by physicians.

Recent studies have even shown its efficacy against MRSA (methicillin-resistant *Staphylococcus aureus*) and other bacteria that were previously resistant to multiple different antibiotics. It is still used currently to treat topical infections and burns to prevent subsequent infections with bacteria and other microorganisms.

The topical preparation is very effective and is known as Silvadene cream or silver sulfadiazine. Silver is also wisely incorporated into a number of wound dressings in order to exploit its antimicrobial activity.

The big fear often cited by many medical "authorities" is a complication of colloidal silver use known as argyria. Argyria is a condition where your skin is permanently dyed blue to blue gray in color. Patients familiar with the work of doctors from the medical underground have been using it for decades, with absolutely no evidence of argyria as a complication. I have many patients who have used small quantities of colloidal silver for years without this complication.

Many patients make their own colloidal silver by using small machines known as colloidal silver generators. I prefer to buy the premixed colloidal silver preparations. For years, I have been using a product known as MesoSilver made by Purest Colloids.

MesoSilver is 20 ppm or parts per million of silver. The committee that studies the use of medicinal silver preparations is known as the Silver Safety Committee. It is composed of physicians and scientists who specialize in the medicinal use of silver preparations.

They have a simple formula for determining the maximum quantity of silver that you can ingest in a day. The formula is your weight in pounds multiplied by 12; the total is then divided by the ppm of the silver preparation, which in the case of Mesosilver is 20.

The answer to that formula is the maximum number of drops of colloidal silver you can safely take in a day. Of course, you don't have to take that much for it to work, especially for GI infections where it appears to be particularly effective. What I would advise is taking it in divided doses three or four times a day until your symptoms have resolved.

Another very effective way to treat GI infections that are causing diarrhea is to use mucilaginous herbs. Mucilaginous herbs are herbs that form into a slippery gel-like consistency when they are mixed with water.

I have found three different mucilaginous herbs to be very useful in the treatment of diarrhea—they are psyllium husk or seed (*Plantago ovata*), slippery elm (*Ulmus fulva*) and marshmallow root (*Althea officinalis*). All three of these work in similar ways. They contain large amounts of soluble fiber that absorbs water and thus helps decrease diarrhea.

In addition to which, they coat and soothe the irritated, infected intestinal lining. By their actions, they bind up toxins and carry them away from the intestine, hence decreasing inflammation, promoting its healing.

My favorite of the three is slippery elm, which also has excellent nutritional content, thus helping someone who has had prolonged diarrhea. You should note that since all three of these mucilaginous herbs have outstanding absorptive capacity, you should not take any medications two hours before or after using them (just like activated charcoal).

THE DOSING OF THE THREE MUCILAGINOUS HERBS

Psyllium husk or seed. One teaspoon mixed into a large glass of water three times daily until healed.

Marshmallow root. Make a tea with one teaspoon of it in its powder form in a mug of boiling water, then allow it to steep for ten minutes before drinking it. Drink that tea three times a day as needed until the diarrhea passes.

Slippery elm. Make a porridge by mixing one tablespoon into a mug of hot water; wait for it to cool. It also comes in a tincture, in which case, use 5 mg TID (three times daily) or in convenient 500 mg capsules also TID.

CHAPTER ELEVEN

INFECTIONS OF THE EYE

As you have no doubt noticed earlier in this book, I always like to teach my readers the anatomy of a particular part of the body. In order that they may better understand what can go wrong with it when infected.

The front of the human eye is covered by a clear dome-like surface called the cornea. The cornea lies directly on top of the iris or the part of the eye that gives it its color, such as brown, blue, green, or hazel. I have seen patients with different color irises. This is merely a genetic variation and has no impact upon the function of their eyes.

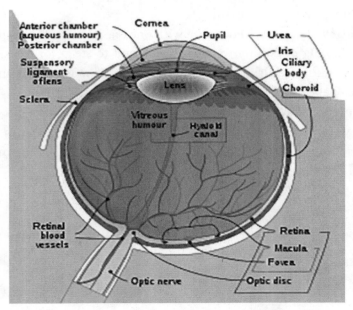

Anatomy of a human eye, compliments of *Wikipedia*.

Light passes through the clear cornea and through the pupil. Directly behind the pupil is the lens. The size of the pupil is controlled by a muscle and some connective tissue known as the iris. If the iris contracts or tightens, this partially closes the pupil, making it smaller, thus allowing less light to enter the eye. This happens when you are outside in bright sunlight, your pupils are very small and pinpoint.

Conversely, when you are inside in a dark room, your iris relaxes. This dilates the pupil, enlarging it, thus allowing more light to enter your eye, helping your vision in the dark. This changing of the amount of light entering your eye by your pupils is known as the pupillary light reflex, and it is what a doctor is checking when we shine lights into your eyes during a physical exam.

The pupils therefore control the amount of light striking the lens of the eye and passing through, entering the interior of the eye. The interior of the eye is made up of a clear jellylike substance known as the vitreous. This beam of light focused by the lens crosses the vitreous and strikes the nerve layer at the back of the eye or retina.

The nerves of the retina create impulses of light, dark, and color that are transmitted to the optic nerve (which lies directly behind the retina) and from there are carried to the brain.

There is a small area within the center of the retina called the macula, which contains light-sensitive cells that help sharpen our visual acuity by increasing our discernment of fine details.

The area of the brain where these impulses are assembled and interpreted into images or vision is known as the visual cortex. It is where our vision is produced for the brain.

One last part of the eye that I need to mention is the conjunctiva. The conjunctiva is a membrane that lines your eyelids and also covers the white part of your eye or sclera. The muscles that move the eye are attached to the sclera.

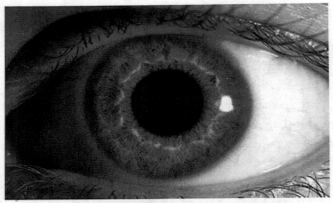

INFECTIONS OF THE EYE

CONJUNCTIVITIS

The most common infection of the eye is conjunctivitis or pink eye. It is the eye infection most often seen in a primary care setting. As you recall, the conjunctiva lines the eyelid and covers the white sclera of your eye, hence even for a layman, it is very easy to identify.

There are three types of conjunctivitis, only two are infectious: bacterial and viral. The third type is allergic conjunctivitis, and this is not caused by an infection but, as the name implies, by allergies. Hence it is not contagious like the other two and cannot be transmitted to others.

All three have symptoms in common such as swollen eyelids, red eyes, glassy-appearing eyes, a gritty feeling to the eye, blurry vision at times, burning, and itching.

The name pink eye tells it all—your eye's white part or sclera is reddened and often tearing. Pink eye is caused by infections that are either bacterial or viral in origin. They can be distinguished by the type of discharge they produce.

If it is a thick yellow/green sticky discharge and you find your eyelids lined with this goop upon awakening in the morning, then you have a bacterial infection. This pustular discharge or goop, as patients like to call it, will often form strings hanging from your eyelids. On the other hand, if it produces a thin watery clear or sometimes white discharge, then it is most likely viral in origin.

Not to further confuse matters but allergic conjunctivitis also produces a thin watery discharge but is accompanied by allergy-related problems such as sneezing, nasal congestion, etc.

Conjunctivitis, either bacterial or viral, is highly contagious and easily spread to the uninfected eye by hand-to-eye contact. If you have it long enough, you will invariably spread it to your healthy eye.

I always advise patients to try not to touch their eyes and to frequently wash their hands to prevent transmission. But do they listen? Hell no, and of course they not only spread it to their good eye but also transmit the infection to others via doorknobs, handshaking, and countless other ways. And thus the infection continues on and on among the human population.

I often wonder if an infection like conjunctivitis latched onto some unfortunate human thousands of years ago and has remained unchanged, continuously infecting mankind ever since. I don't know the answer to that, but the thought intrigues me.

TREATMENT OF CONJUNCTIVITIS

The good news is that conjunctivitis is usually self-limited and will run its course and eventually be healed by the body. Usually, in a week or two, it will be gone. However, that being said, I would treat it as soon as possible, both for personal relief as well as to halt its spread.

Here are some general principles of treatment for all types of conjunctivitis. First of all, *do not rub your eyes, and touch them as little as possible*. Trust me—that is not an easy thing to do. Wash your hands with soap and water every few hours while awake. If you have contacts, take them out until the conjunctivitis is healed.

Hard contacts should be disinfected for at least twelve hours before using them again. You might want to use a pair of glasses instead of your contacts for a week or two, just to prevent mechanically irritating the surface of your eyes.

Throw away your eye makeup; it is likely contaminated. Change your pillowcase and sheets daily, if possible, especially the pillowcase as it is very likely heavily contaminated.

You should keep your eyes well lubricated. The last thing you want is a dry, gritty eye. Use artificial tears or some of the other eyewashes I am going to show you below.

If your eyes hurt and/or are swollen, then you need to apply cold compresses. You can do this as often as you like, but usually three or four times a day suffices. Take a facecloth or small towel, soak it in very cold water, gently wring it out, and then apply across both of your eyes (while lying down). A cold pack of any type or ice pack will work even better. It will also help any frontal sinus–type headache.

You should also clean your eyes to remove any discharge. There is no point in leaving it to dry and stick to your eyelid. The easiest way to clean your eyes is with a warm, wet face cloth. Wipe from the medial side of your eye (the side closest to your nose), towards the outside.

EYEWASHES

If you have conjunctivitis, you will need to flush out your eyes periodically with an eyewash. What this does is remove any irritants or allergens if you have allergic conjunctivitis. Or if your eyes have been irritated by some foreign substance like a strong soap, an eyewash will flush your eyes, eliminating it.

The benefits of lubricating your eyes with an eyewash should not be underestimated. Many of the eyewashes I am going to describe, also have antibacterial and/or antiviral actions. These can either be applied with an eye dropper, or you can use an eyecup. Flushing out your infected eyes with an eyewash will help flush away bacteria and pus and other debris from the infection and is the only way to effectively treat infectious conjunctivitis or pink eye.

1. *Aloe vera*. Aloe vera has so many uses in general, but for eye infections, it is especially useful since it is antibacterial, antifungal, and antiviral. Take fresh aloe vera juice and instill two drops in each infected eye three times a day. It is incredibly soothing as well as a potent disinfectant.

2. *Milk and honey*. Take two cups of milk, bring it to a boil, and then dissolve three teaspoons of honey into it while stirring it constantly in order to properly combine the two. Allow it to cool down and then using a clean eyedropper (squirt a few streams of boiling water thru it to clean it), apply two or three drops into each eye every four to six hours.

3. *Lemon juice*. Take a lemon and squeeze a few drops of its juice into some warm water and use this to gently wash or flush out your eyes. Do not use it without diluting it. Use several drops three or four times a day to soothe and flush your eyes.

4. *Salt water or saline solution*. You can make your own saline solution by mixing one teaspoon of salt, either table or sea salt, in one cup of distilled water. Bring this mix to a boil, allow it to cool down (isn't it pitiful that I have to say that), and use it to flush out your eye, either with an eye dropper or with an eyecup.

5. *Baking soda*. Same as above, mix one tablespoon of baking soda in two cups of distilled water. Boil the mix and allow it to cool and use it liberally to flush out your eyes.

6. *Boric acid*. All pharmacies have this; it is over-the-counter and does not require a prescription. Boric acid is made from borax and is a weak acid crystalline powder. It is very inexpensive and very effective against eye infections since it is also an antiseptic. Mix one teaspoon of boric acid in a cup of water, bring it to a boil, allow it to cool. Soak some cotton balls into the solution and apply them to your eyes or make an eyewash using an eyecup and flush out the infected eyes with it. Afterward, flush out your eyes with lukewarm water to eliminate any residue. Use boric acid three or four times a day until the infection is resolved.

7. *Calendula*. Calendula is an herb that has both very potent antibacterial and antiviral properties. In addition, it is very soothing to the eye. This combination makes it an excellent choice for eye infections. Take two teaspoons of dried calendula flowers and put them in a cup of water and brew a tea from them. After bringing it to a boil, allow it to cool. Using a coffee filter or cheesecloth, strain it to remove any particulate matter

(junk floating in it). Using an eyecup, apply it several times a day until you are fully healed.

8. Eyebright or *Euphrasia officinalis*: This herb has been in use since the time of the Romans. Take one teaspoon of the dried herb and mix in it one cup of water and bring it to a boil; allow it to cool. Filter out any particulate matter with a coffee filter or cheesecloth. Use the liquid with an eyecup up to four times a day until your infection is healed. It can also be made into warm compresses by soaking a small piece of cloth in it and applying it over both closed eyes.

9. *Chamomile.* Chamomile is a flower in the Aster family. It is prepared exactly as eyebright in the previous paragraph. You should note that if you use teabags for any of the above preparations, you can use those bags topically over your closed eyes to soothe them. After which, toss them into your compost pile. Never waste anything if you can help it. Tea bags and coffee grinds are full of minerals and plant nutrients and are wonderful soil amendments.

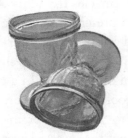

Eyecups used to irrigate your eyes.

10. *Cucumber.* This one is a little more complicated than the other treatments on this list. First, you must make sure your hands are really clean, even under your fingernails. Wash them thoroughly with soap and water. Also clean the outside of the cucumber, also with soap and water and rinse it well. Take a raw cucumber, peel, and grate it. Take a large sterile gauze pad or cheesecloth (that has been boiled to sterilize it) and fill it with the cucumber.

11. *Povidone-iodine solution (Betadine).* Here I saved the best and most effective treatment for last. None of the previous

treatments I mentioned on this list come close to the killing power of Betadine for bacterial, fungal, and viral eye infections.

As I have mentioned many times earlier in this book, iodine is universally deadly to all pathogens. It is even deadly to MRSA and tuberculosis infections. The strength Betadine you should use is 5 percent as stronger versions might cause burning to your eyes. If you have a stronger version, dilute it down with water to 5 percent or less. You can use an eyedropper to place a drop or two in each eye. Do this twice a day until the infection is resolved.

Once you put the drops in, take a few seconds to rotate each eye to spread the Betadine over your eye surface. Look up as far as you can then down, then left and right; that should coat it completely. It might discolor the white part or sclera of your eye yellow/brown for a few days, but it will eventually wash away. Betadine should not be used if you are allergic to iodine or are pregnant.

OTHER EYE INFECTIONS: STYES, BLEPHARITIS, CHALAZION, AND HORDEOLUMS

Let me first clarify the differences between all the above terms. The general public calls a red swelling at the edge of the eyelid a stye. The medical term for which is a hordeolum. It typically involves the base of the hairs of the eyelid and the meibomian glands, which are oil glands that lubricate them.

These hordeolum can cause swelling and redness to the eyelid, sometimes diffuse (spread out), other times a small round swelling. The vast majority of these hordeolum are caused by the bacteria *Staph. aureus*. These can be treated with warm compresses four times a day. I would also clean the external eye with betadine (5 percent) twice a day until it is resolved. You can also clean the lid with baby shampoo or liquid soap twice a day, but I find Betadine to be infinitely more effective.

If the infection involves the entire edge of the eyelids rather than a small area like a stye, then it is known as blepharitis. Although that being said, there are times when blepharitis causes swelling of the entire eyelid. The treatment is the same, using hot compresses four times a day and either Betadine, baby shampoo, or liquid soap to clean the lids and keep them free of pustular debris and all that eye goop.

Sometimes an eye infection will form a chalazion. A chalazion is a small, usually hard area of swelling and redness to the eyelid. It is caused by the blockage of a sebaceous gland and the resulting formation of a granuloma. It is a chronic condition and oftentimes painless. They are treated just like the conditions above—that is with hot compresses four times daily, cleansing the lid with either Betadine, Ivory soap, or baby shampoo. Since chalazions are a chronic condition, it might take up to a few weeks of treatment to reverse and heal them.

If the eyeball itself gets irritated while you have any of the abovenamed conditions, then you may use one of the many effective eyewashes that I named earlier. My personal choice would be the Betadine.

Finally, I would like to mention that if you have swelling of your eyelids, there are a variety of topical treatments that will give you some relief. Ice packs or cold compresses of any type are very effective at bringing down swelling. Applying cucumber slices, tea bags, potato slices, or any cold fruit packed into a pair of old ski goggles will work just fine. I did that once in medical school using watermelon, and it worked like a charm. Be creative—think outside the box and you might just surprise yourself with a novel effective treatment.

CHAPTER TWELVE

THE HORROR OF CHRONIC INFECTIONS

What if many of the infections we had in the past never totally healed and are still present in many of our body's tissues, leading to many of the allergies, autoimmune dysfunction, chronic diseases, and even cancer that so many of us currently suffer with?

We all tend to think infections start with one or more heralding symptoms and progress until eradicated by either our immune systems or combined with modern therapeutics such as antibiotics, antiviral, and antifungal medications.

There is now mounting evidence that many, if not most, infections have a second phase where the surviving pathogens establish colonies within our bodies. They are able to do so only by evading detection by the immune system. Since if they were detected, there would be an ever-increasing immune response and many accompanying symptoms such as fever, muscle aches, diaphoresis (sweating), headache, and gastrointestinal problems.

Think of it this way, if you are an invading germ, your best option is to become stealthy and make yourself invisible to all of the body's sophisticated mechanisms of detection. They do this by making a dome or biofilm over the survivors of the original infection.

This biofilm acts as a cloaking device, rendering the colony it covers invisible to the host's immune system. It does this by presenting proteins on its surface that are not recognized as foreign, but rather as "self." Thus the pathogens can thrive below in their own little colony unmolested by all the passing scavengers of the immune system, who for all intents and purposes have no clue they are there.

These pathologic biofilm colonies have been named chronic pathogen colonization or CPC by Dr. Thomas E. Levy in his most recent fascinating book entitled *Rapid Virus Recovery*.

Dr. Levy is a brilliant physician who is clearly part of what I like to call the medical underground. He is an independent thinker and a pioneer in many of his medical treatments. He has been fighting the good fight for vitamin C for many decades, demonstrating its endless medical applications in treating many diseases. He especially highlights vitamin C as a nontoxic, inexpensive, readily available potent antiviral, capable of eradicating all viral infections. He has written a host of outstanding books, each heavily researched and documented, that I highly recommend.

What if—there were very few, if any—past infections that your body had completely eradicated? What if most of your past infections had survivors who have remained protected, undetected, thriving under their biofilms? That second stealth phase of chronic infection by CPC is not on the radar of mainstream medicine.

For physicians, the general assumption is that if we treat an infection and the symptoms resolve and all vital signs return to normal, then we won and our job is done. As it turns out, there is mounting evidence of the persistence of many infections and hence the presence of these colonies in most people.

CPC are in many parts of our respiratory system since that is the most frequently infected part of the body, which is due to the amazing volume of air that crosses it daily. That outside air at times is teeming with respiratory pathogens just hankering for some good respiratory tract cells to land on.

Consequently, CPC form most commonly in our gums, teeth, nose, sinuses, tonsils, and lungs. How bad could that be? you naively ask. Aha, my little grasshopper, let me put it succinctly: it is a grave disaster for your health.

These pathogenic (disease causing) colonies lead to chronic infections such as *Helicobacter pylori* in your stomach, *Candida albicans*, SIBO (small intestinal bacterial overgrowth), chronic Lyme disease, MRSA (methicillin resistant *Staph. aureus*), periodontal disease, chronic ear and sinus infections, inflammatory skin infections such as seborrheic dermatitis and atopic dermatitis, chronic skin infections like athlete's foot, onychomycosis or chronic fungal infections of finger and toenails, indwelling catheter infections, infections of implants, endocarditis, and chronic wound infections to name but a few.

In addition to which, many parasites also chronically colonize our bodies, especially our GI tract.

The problem is that these colonies release a steady stream of waste products and toxins along with pathogenic (disease causing) members of their colony into both the venous and lymphatic circulations. Hence they constantly seed the host's body with a devil's brew that it must detoxify and sterilize.

This in turn occupies your immune system with constant invaders, burdens your liver with detoxification, and damages the GI tracts intestinal flora or microbiome as well as damaging the enterocytes that line the gut. These enterocytes are normally jammed shoulder to shoulder in a single file, lining the gut.

Once they are damaged, gaps develop between the enterocytes, thus allowing large proteins or pieces of protein to penetrate the gut lining and enter into the bloodstream. This condition is appropriately named leaky gut syndrome. It in turn is thought to be the cause of the autoimmune diseases, allergies of all types commonly including food allergies.

It also is a very likely source for most of our chronic diseases and even cancer. However, leaky gut syndrome is not recognized by mainstream medicine, nor do they have a cause for the explosion of allergies, autoimmune and chronic diseases. Once again, the medical underground mobilizes and finds plausible answers to these medical mysteries.

Chronic infections, as I alluded to earlier, are biphasic, meaning they have two phases. Phase 1 is the initial infection. This initial infection is defeated by the body but, unfortunately, many times, not totally eradicated. Small pockets of pathogens from the original infection are able to survive by creating biofilm domes over themselves and thriving within them.

Phase 2 begins once the biofilm protective layer is made. Now the colonies are festering within the biofilm and are producing waste products and toxins that constantly attack our bodies, causing inflammation and tissue damage with the results being chronic diseases such as arthritis, hypertension (high blood pressure), diabetes, autoimmune diseases, chronic allergies, and inflammatory bowel diseases such as Crohn's disease and ulcerative colitis to name but a few.

If that wasn't horrible enough, often bacteria, viruses, and fungi also escape the biofilm colonies and spread to other parts of the body.

Since the primary portal of entry for most germs is via our respiratory system, that is where most chronic infections get established. Many others also get established in our gastrointestinal tract, which is the second most common site of infections.

Hence that is where we must concentrate our efforts to eradicate chronic infections. Mind you, this is no easy task. Chronic infections require chronic treatment to suppress them and hopefully eradicate them.

TREATMENT OF CHRONIC INFECTIONS

In order to treat chronic infections, essentially what we need to do is unravel or reverse the original process from which they began. Therefore we need to focus our initial treatments on the respiratory tract, starting in the nose, sinuses, mouth, pharynx, throat, and lungs.

As I have said for many years, I have never seen a patient with bad teeth in good health; the two just don't go together. Your health begins in your mouth simply because that is where chronic periodontal infections and, ultimately, chronic disease states begin.

Oral plaque and tartar are the observable manifestations of biofilm growth in our mouths. These biofilms form on the surface of teeth both above and below the gumline. They also form on the tongue, gums, and the inside of our cheeks. The longer these CPC remain in your mouth, the more damage they will cause.

These oral biofilm colonies or CPC cause several stages of disease involving the gums, teeth, and jawbone. Chronic infections from biofilm on teeth begin on the tooth surface above the gumline and eventually migrate below the gumline. This in turn leads to inflammation of the gums, which in its early stages is known as gingivitis.

Healthy gums should be snug around your teeth, pink in color, and not sensitive to touch. Symptoms of gingivitis include red, inflamed-appearing gums that bleed easily with brushing or flossing of your teeth and may also be painful. These are all warning signs of gum disease.

The second stage of gum disease is periodontitis. Periodontitis is a much more serious gum infection that both damages the gums as well as the bone in which the teeth are imbedded. This will lead to retraction of the gums and loosening of the teeth, eventually allowing them to fall out.

Periodontal disease is widespread in the United States. A recent report by the CDC said that 47.2 percent of Americans over thirty had periodontal disease, and that number rose to 70.1 percent for the elderly (older than sixty-five).

When you have periodontal disease and you brush your teeth, it will cause pathogenic or disease-causing bacteria to enter your blood and travel to your heart, lungs, and many other areas of your body, leading to infections and inflammation throughout your body and, in turn, many if not most chronic diseases.

How common are chronic diseases in the United States? United States government statistics report that 51 percent of Americans suffer with at least one chronic disease such as arthritis, diabetes, hypertension, asthma, heart disease, stroke, cancer, and chronic respiratory disease.

Even more horrifying is that 26 percent of Americans have multiple chronic diseases! What is mainstream medicine doing about it? We are throwing billions of dollars of toxic pharmaceuticals at the problem. We are beating up people about their poor diets, lack of exercise, and bad habits like smoking, drinking, and recreational drug abuse.

While all these are important factors in helping address chronic diseases, they simply are not working. The United States population and those of most of the world are becoming progressively more obese, sedentary, and disease ridden. Almost a century of our efforts to stem and reverse these chronic diseases has been an abysmal failure.

If you want to eliminate and reverse these chronic diseases, we must first treat the chronic underlying infections. In my not so humble opinion, that is the most practical way forward. In addition to which, our medical underground methods help detoxify and support your body and do not have the harmful side effects associated with the handful of pills mainstream medicine is currently offering us.

To my mind, that is clearly a win-win situation, and I prefer that to the use of toxic chemicals to treat an already toxic problem!

Okay, let's get started. Your first step has to be to go to your dentist. Any rotten teeth need to be removed, any that can be saved should be. You also need to have twice yearly extensive dental cleaning done by a dental hygienist. This cleaning will remove the plaque that builds up on teeth, discoloring them. These are essentially dental biofilm colonies.

From these colonies, the usual suspects of waste products, toxins and pathogens are swallowed and gain access to the gastrointestinal system. Hence we need to sever that connection—that is why treating the respiratory tract and is so critical to our success.

Between cleanings, you can do your part with regular brushing of your teeth, flossing, and in addition to which, after a good brushing, gargle with a 50 percent mixture (half water mixed with half peroxide, for those of you of who are math-challenged) of hydrogen peroxide and water.

This will allow the peroxide to penetrate into all the nooks and crannies of your mouth to kill any residual germs. You can also use a Waterpik machine with hydrogen peroxide at 3 percent to rinse deeply between your teeth. If done correctly, it is less traumatic to the gums than flossing, and more effective.

If done routinely, your dental hygienist will remark as mine did that you have not produced hardly any plague since your last cleaning. Gargling with the half-peroxide-and-water mix will also help clean your oral pharynx and the upper part of your throat and help prevent colonization of your tonsils.

This regimen of gargling and rinsing out your mouth will also greatly reduce the number of upper respiratory tract infections such as the common cold. There is no real downside to it; hydrogen peroxide is very inexpensive and readily available.

You may want to purchase food-grade hydrogen peroxide in order to avoid any chemical stabilizers in store-bought hydrogen peroxide.

However, they are arguably most likely negligible in their impact, but better to not have them if possible.

If you do so, it will need to be diluted down to minimum of 3 percent, which is the same as store-bought hydrogen peroxide. For our purposes, we will dilute it with normal saline solution for nebulization; for gargling, you can dilute it with water.

For our purposes, in order to eliminate CPC, I recommend using 3 percent hydrogen peroxide to start with. If you experience any burning sensation from it, dilute it in half to 1.5 percent by mixing an equal amount of saline into the 3 percent solution.

That being said, 3 percent is usually very well tolerated and does not require further dilution, but some patients are very sensitive. I would also recommend using a facial mask with your nebulizer instead of a mouthpiece. This will also treat your nose and sinuses instead of your mouth and parts below. As always, everything is available on Amazon.

The frequency of your nebulizer treatments with hydrogen peroxide varies, depending on the severity of your illness. If you have an acute infection superimposed on your chronic disease state, then you should nebulize three or four times a day.

Once your acute symptoms are resolved, continue this high frequency for another three days, just to insure adequate eradication. Then step it down to once or twice a day, depending on the severity of your health. The first thing you will notice is that your bowels will heal.

Once your periodontal disease and other upper and lower respiratory tract diseases are cured, then the steady stream of disease-causing toxins will also disappear. Once this happens, the gut-lining cells or enterocytes will heal; and in turn, your leaky gut syndrome will also heal.

You can help your gut heal by also using probiotics with prebiotics to feed them. I would also include fermented foods of all types in your diet to further provide healthy probiotics, enzymes, minerals, and thus further support for your gut microbiome.

Examples of good, fermented foods that support gut health include sauerkraut, yogurt, kefir, kombucha, kimchi, tempeh, and miso.

Remember that the hydrogen peroxide nebulizer treatments are infinitely more effective when combined with other supportive therapies such as the gang of seven. The only way to have any chance of eradication of these chronic infections is to hit them on every level, thus the importance of chronically taking the gang of seven along with nebulization.

All the gang of seven components are essential especially vitamin C. Severe illnesses consume massive amounts of vitamin C, oftentimes inducing clinical scurvy. I would recommend a minimum of two grams of vitamin C daily as a starting point.

Ideally, the highest dose you can tolerate is the best dose for you. It is completely nontoxic and safe. If you develop diarrhea, lower the dose or change to the liposomal vitamin C.

Some medical underground doctors are using very effective treatments such as intravenous hydrogen peroxide, intravenous vitamin C, intravenous magnesium chloride, hyperbaric oxygen treatments, and even blood extraction and treatment with ultraviolet light irradiation and or ozone.

Unfortunately, there are very few doctors who are offering these treatments currently, but they are extremely effective. These medical underground treatments appear to have greater cure rates than simply nebulizing hydrogen peroxide and associated oral treatments.

The take-home message is the greater the number of ways you can support your immune system along with hydrogen peroxide nebulization, the greater your long-term success at healing these chronic infections. My take-home message to you is to be patient.

You presumably have had these chronic infections for quite some time, they have a firm foothold in your body, and it will take some time to eradicate them completely. Not all chronic infections will be healed by any single or combination of therapies, but these treatments from the medical underground are certainly your best hope at treating them.

REFERENCES

Note: I did not give page numbers or chapter numbers to coincide with my use of the below references since many of them were used repeatedly throughout the book. Instead, I will list them by subject matter, not by author.

"6 Benefits of Reishi Mushroom (Plus Side Effects and Dosage)." Grant Tinsley, Ph.D. March 31, 2018. Healthline.

"23 Effective Home Remedies for Skin Infection." Ramona Sipha. January, 9, 2020. Stylecraze.com.

Acquiring Genomes: A Theory of the Origins of Species. Lynn Margulis and Dorion Sagan. 2002. Basic Books.

An Alternative Approach to Allergies: The New Field of Clinical Ecology Unravels the Environmental Causes of Mental and Physical Ills. Theron G. Randolph, MD and Ralph W. Moss, PhD. Revised edition 1989. Harper Row Publishers.

An Epidemic of Absence: A New Way of Understanding Allergies and Autoimmune Disease. Moises Velasquez-Manoff. 2012. Scribner.

"Another Reason to Add Quercetin to Your Daily Supplements." Dr. Joseph Mercola. February 2, 2020. Mercola.com

"Antifungal Mechanisms supporting Boric Acid therapy of Candida vaginitis." De Seta, Schmidt, Vu, Essman, and Larsen. December 2008. *Journal of Antimicrobial Chemotherapy.*

Anti-Inflammatory Oxygen Therapy. Dr. Marc Sircus. 2015. Square One Publishers.

Ascorbate: The Science of Vitamin C. Dr. Steve Hickey and Dr. Hilary Roberts. Self-published, 2004.

"Assessment of Helicobacter pylori Eradication by Virgin Olive Oil." Castro et al. August 2012.

"Asymptomatic 'Casedemic' Is a Perpetuation of Needless Fear." Dr. Joseph Mercola. November 24, 2020. Mercola.com.

"Asymptomatic People Do Not Spread COVID-19." Dr. Joseph Mercola. December 7, 2020. Mercola.com.

The Autoimmune Fix. Dr. Tom O'Bryan. 2016. Rodale Books.

"Avoid Serious Complications from Viral Infections." Dr. Marc Sircus. www.DrSircus.com.

Baking Soda: Over 500 Fabulous, Fun, and Frugal Uses You've Probably Never Thought Of. Vicki Lasnky. 2004. Book Peddlers.

"Best Nutrients for Cold and Flu Season." Dr. Joseph Mercola. October 31, 2018. Mercola.com.

Biochemical Individuality: The Key to Understanding What Is Shaping Your Health. Roger J. Williams PhD. 1956. John Wiley and Sons.

Biological Inorganic Chemistry: A New Introduction to Molecular Structure and Function. Robert R. Crichton. 2008. Elsevier.

The Body Electric: Electromagnetism and the Foundation of Life. Robert O. Becker, MD and Gary Selden. 1985. William Morrow and Company.

"Bromelain as a Proteolytic Enzyme." Sherril Sego. Clinical Advisor. June 3, 2016.

Cancer and Vitamin C: A Discussion of the Nature, Causes, Prevention and Treatment of Cancer with Special Reference to the Value of Vitamin C. Linus Pauling and Ewan Cameron. 1979. W. W. Norton and Company.

Cancer is a Fungus: A Revolution in Tumor Therapy. Dr. T. Simoncini. 2005. Edizioni Lampis.

Cancer and the New Biology of Water. Dr. Thomas Cowan. 2019. Chelsea Green publisher.

"Can Face Masks Protect You from Aerosol Particles? An interview with Denis Rancourt." Mercola.com.

"CDC Caught Cooking the Books on COVID Vaccines." Dr. Joseph Mercola. June 17, 2021. Mercola.com.

"CDC Scandal: Committee that Withdrew Recommendation for Nasal Flu Vaccine Now Recommends It to Experiment on American Public." March 19, 2018. Health Impact News.

"Characteristics of Traditional Diets." by Jill Nienhiser, January 1, 2000. Weston A. Price Foundation. www.WESTONAPRICE.ORG/AUTHOR/NIENHISER

Charcoal Remedies. John Dinsley. 2005. Gatekeeper Books. charcoalremedies.com

The Chemistry of Essential Oils Made Simple: God's Love Manifest in Molecules. David Stewart. 2010, 3rd printing. Care Publications.

"Chromium." National Institute of Health website.

"Chromium." WebMd.com.

Clinical Nutrition of the Essential Trace Elements and Minerals: The Guide for Health Professionals. edited by John D. Bogden, PhD and Leslie M. Klevay, MD. 2000. Human Press Publishers.

Colloidal Minerals and Trace Elements: How to Restore the Body's Natural Vitality. M. Muller, MD, ND, and PhD. 2002. Healing Arts Press.

Complete Book of Minerals for Health. J. I. Rodale and staff. 1967, 6th printing. Rodale Books.

"Copper's Virus-killing Powers Were Known Even to the Ancients." Jim Morrison. April 14, 2020. *Smithsonian Magazine.*

"Coronavirus: Early Research Provides Hope that One Supplement Could Help Control It—Quercetin." March 27, 2020. Institute for Natural Healing. institutefornaturalhealing.com.

"Could Hydrogen Peroxide Treat Coronavirus?" Dr. Joseph Mercola. April 10, 2020. Mercola.com.

"Could Mouthwash Be an Ally in fighting COVID-19?" Dr. Joseph Mercola. June 15, 2020. Mercola.com.

"COVID-19 Critical Care." Front Line COVID-19 Critical Care Working Group. June 1, 2020. Mercola.com.

"COVID-19: How Can I Cure Thee? Let Me Count the Ways." Dr. Thomas E. Levy. Orthomolecular News Service. July 18, 2020.

"COVID-19 Testing Scandal Deepens." Dr. Joseph Mercola. December 28, 2020. Mercola.com.

"COVID Conflicts: Asymptomatic Testing, Lack of Danger to Kids." Dr. Joseph Mercola. December 31, 2020. Mercola.com.

"Covid, Ivermectin, and the Crime of the Century." Bret Weinstein, PhD. June 17, 2021. Mercola.com.

"Covid Vaccines May Bring an Avalanche of Neurological Disease: An interview with Stephanie Seneff, PhD." MIT. May 24, 2021. Mercola.com.

"COVID-19 vs. Homo Sapiens Ascorbicus." Theo Farmer. November 20, 2020. Orthomolecular Medicine News Service.

Curing the Incurable: Vitamin C Infectious Disease and Toxins. Thomas E. Levy. 2009 3rd Edition. LivOn Books.

"Curing Viruses with Hydrogen Peroxide: Can a Simple Therapy Stop the Pandemic?" Thomas E. Levy, MD, JD. August 21, 2020. Orthomolecular Medicine News Service.

"The Dangerous Way Flu Symptoms are Disguised in Older Adults." Joyce Hoffman: February 25, 2018. Easyhealthoptions.com.

"The Dangers of Root Canals and How to Treat Them." Dr. Joseph Mercola. April 12, 2021. Mercola.com.

Dead Doctors Don't Lie. Dr. Joel D. Wallach and Dr. Ma Lan. 1999. Wellness Publications LLC.

The Decline of the World's IQ. Richard Lynn and John Harvey. March–April 2008. Intelligence.

Deep Nutrition: Why Your Genes Need Traditional Food. Catherine W. Shanahan MD and Luke Shanahan. 2009. Big Box Books.

Degeneration, Regeneration. Melvin E. Page, DDS 1949. Biochemical Research Foundation.

DHA: The Magnificent Marine Oil (Health Learning Handbook). Beth M. Ley-Jacobs, PhD. 1999. BL Publications

"Did This Scientist Develop a Cure for COVID-19? An interview with Jacob Glanville, PhD." April 21, 2020. Mercola.com.

"The Different Forms of Vitamin E: In Depth Research on Essential Vitamins." Dr. George Obiikoya. Vitamins-Nutrition.org.

The Disease Delusion: Conquering the Causes of Chronic Illness for a Healthier, Longer, and Happier Life. Dr. Jeffrey Bland. 2014. HarperCollins Books.

Disease Prevention and Treatment. Life Extension Foundation, Expanded 4th edition, 2003. Life Extension Media.

"Does Zinc Supplementation Enhance the Clinical Efficacy of Chloroquine and Hydroxychloroquine to win todays battle against COVID-19." Derwand and Schotz. May 2020. Medical Hypotheses.

Dr. Mark Stengler's Natural Healing Library. Dr. Mark Stengler. 2011. Bottom Line Books.

The Doomsday Book of Medicine. Dr. Ralph La Guardia. 2015. Mindstir Media.

"Dosages and Treatments for Coronavirus Infections." Dr. Marc Sircus. www.DrSircus.com.

"Effects of Chromium on the Immune System." Shrivastava et al. Volume 34, issue 1; September 2002. FEMS Immunology and Medical Microbiology.

"The Effects of Iodine on Intelligence in Children; a metanalyses of studies conducted in China." M. Qian MD et al. September 10, 2004. Asia Pacific Journal of Clinical Nutrition.

"The Effects of Vitamin D and Covid-Related Questions." Dr. Joseph Mercola. July 9, 2021. Mercola.com.

Empty Harvest: Understanding the Link between our Food, our Immunity and our Planet. Dr. Bernard Jensen and Mark Anderson. 1990. Avery Publishing Group.

Energy Medicine: The Scientific Basis. James L. Oschman. 2000. Churchill Livingstone Books.

Enzymes: The Key to Health, Volume I (The Fundamentals). Howard F. Loomis Jr. DC. 2012. American Printing Company, Inc.

Enzymes: What the Experts Know; The Role of Enzyme Therapy in Restoring, Promoting and Maintaining Optimal Health. Tom Bohager. 2006. One World Press.

"Essential Nutrition to Protect Yourself from Coronavirus." Dr. Joseph Mercola. March 10, 2020. Mercola.com.

"Estimating or Measuring? What Is the True Effect of Vitamin D on Covid-19?" Robert G. Smith, PhD. June 12, 2021. Orthomolecular Medicine News Service.

The Fast Diet: Lose Weight, Stay Healthy, and Live Longer with the Simple Secret of Intermittent Fasting. Dr. M. Mosley and Mimi Spencer. 2013. Atria Books.

"Fauci Backpedals on Vitamin C and D Recommendations." Dr. Joseph Mercola. April 23, 2020. Mercola.com

Fertility from the Ocean Deep. Charles Walters. 2005. Acres USA.

"Fight Fatigue with Fluids." November 2013. Harvard Health Publishing, Harvard Medical School.

"Flu Vaccine: The Horrible 'Immune System Mistake' Millions Will Make This Year." Dr. Joseph Mercola. February 18, 2016. Mercola.com.

"Forms, Doses, and Effects of Vitamins C and E." Robert G. Smith, PhD. April 27, 2020. Orthomolecular Medicine News Service.

"Former Pfizer Science Officer Reveals Great COVID-19 Scam: An Interview with Michael Yeadon, PhD." December 1, 2020; Mercola.com.

The Fourth Phase of Water: Beyond Solid, Liquid and Vapor. Gerald H. Pollack. 2013. Ebner and Sons Publisher.

The Free Man's Declaration for Health and Longevity. William Campbell Douglas II MD. 2013. New Market Health Publishing.

From Soil to Supplement: A Course in Food, Diet and Nutrition. Dr. Royal Lee. Reprinted 2005. Serene River Press.

"Function and Mechanism of Zinc Metalloenzymes." K. McCall, C. Huang, and Carol A. Fierke. 2000. American Society for Nutritional Sciences.

The Germ that Causes Cancer. Doug A. Kaufmann and Beverly Thornhill Hunt, PhD. 2002. Media Trition.

The Healing Intelligence of Essential Oils: The Science of Advanced Aromatherapy. Kurt Schnabel, PhD. 2011. Healing Arts Press.

The Healing Nutrients Within: Facts, Findings, and New Research on Amino Acids. by Eric. R. Braverman MD with Carl C. Pfeiffer MD. 1987. Keats.

Healing Is Voltage: The Handbook, Third Edition. Jerry Tennant, MD. 2010. CreateSpace Independent publishing platform.

The Healing Power of Fever: Your Body's Natural Defense against Disease. Christopher Vasey MD. 2008. Healing Arts Press

The Healing Sun: Sunlight and Health in the 21ˢᵗ Century. Richard Hobaday PhD. 1999. Findhorn Press.

Healing with Iodine: Your Missing Link to Better Health. Dr. Marc Sircus. 2018. Square One Publishers.

"Chaga." WebMD website.

"A Health Crisis Exposed by the COVID Pandemic." Charles Bens. January 15, 2021. Orthomolecular Medicine News Service.

Health from the Sea and Soil: How to Keep Healthier, Feel Better, and Live Longer Using Nature's Vital Nutrients. Charles B. Ahlson, 1962, Exposition Press.

Health from the Seas: Freedom from Disease. John Croft. 2003. Vital Health Publishing.

"A Healthy Microbiome Builds a Strong Immune System that Could Help Defeat COVID-19." Anna Maldonado-Contreras. January 26, 2021. Theconversation.com.

Helicobacter pylori Treatment: antibiotics or probiotics: by Wojska Polskiego and Kamila Goderska. October 26, 2017. www.ncbi.nlm.nih.gov .

Helping Yourself to Health from the Sea. Howard H. Hirschhorn. 1979. Parker Publishing Company.

"High-Dose Intravenous Vitamin C Treatment for COVID-19." Adnan Erol MD. March 21, 2020. Orthomolecular Medicine News Service.

A Holistic Approach to Viruses. David Brownstein, MD. 2021. Medical Alternatives Press.

"Home Remedies for Skin Infections." No author cited. May 7, 2010. Speedyremedies.com.

"How Changing the Definition of Pandemic Altered Our World." Dr. Joseph Mercola. December 14, 2020. Mercola.com

"How COVID-19 is Changing the Future of Vaccines." Dr. Joseph Mercola. January 13, 2021. Mercola.com.

"How Covid Vaccines Can Cause Blood Clots and More." Dr. Sucharit Bhakdi. June 2021. Doctors for COVID Ethics: in a letter to the European Medicines Agency (EMA).

"How COVID-19 Vaccines Can Destroy Your Immune System." Dr. Joseph Mercola. December 26, 2020. Mercola.com.

"How Long Will We Ignore the Truth About Vitamin D?" Dr. Joseph Mercola. December 14, 2020. Mercola.com.

"How Nebulized Peroxide Helps against Respiratory Infections." An interview with Dr. David Brownstein. December 28, 2020. Mercola.com.

"How Nitric Oxide Combats COVID-19." Dr. Joseph Mercola. October 18, 2020. Mercola.com.

"How Safe Are the Nanoparticles in Moderna's Vaccine?" Dr. Joseph Mercola. February 11, 2021. Mercola.com.

"How the Gut Microbiota Influences Our Immune System." Sarah Adães, PhD. July 8, 2019. Neurohackers, neurohacker.com/Qualia-Mind.

"How to Fix the COVID-19 Crisis in 30 Days." Interview with Dr. Damien Downing. July 10, 2020. Mercola.com.

"How to Improve Zinc Uptake to Boost Immune Health." Dr. Joseph Mercola. April 21, 2020. Mercola.com.

"How Vitamin C and Magnesium Help Reverse Disease and Treat Viral Infections." Joseph Mercola. April 13, 2020. LewRockwell.com, Libertarian Hub.

The Illustrated Encyclopedia of Healing Remedies. C. Norman Shealy, MD. 2002. HarperCollins Publishing.

The Immunity Fix: Strengthen Your Immune System, Fight Off Infections, Reverse Chronic Disease and Live a Healthier Life. Dr. James Dinicolantonio and Siim Land. October 2020. Independently published.

"The Importance of Melatonin for Optimal Health." Dr. Joseph Mercola. February 11, 2020. Mercola.com.

"The Influence of Selenium on Immune Responses." Peter R. Hoffman and Marla J. Berry. November 2008. Mal Nutr Food Res: PubMed.

"Influenza Vaccine Linked to Higher COVID Death Rates." Dr. Joseph Mercola. April 27, 2021. Mercola.com.

"Inhaled Magnesium Sulfate in the Treatment of Acute Asthma." Knightly et al. December 12, 2012. Cochrane Library.

"The Insanity of the PCR Testing Saga." Dr. Joseph Mercola. 2021. Mercola.com.

Iodine: Bringing Back the Universal Medicine. Dr. Marc Sircus. April 3, 2011. www.Dr.Sircus.com.

The Iodine Crisis: What You Don't Know about Iodine Can Wreck Your Life. Lynne Farrow. 2013. Devon Press.

Iodine: Why You Need It, Why You Can't Live without It 3ʳᵈ Edition. David Brownstein, MD. 2008. Medical Alternative Press.

"Iodine Your IQ: Key to Unlocking Your Third Eye." No author cited. January 18, 2017. QuantumStones.com.

"Is Quercetin a Safer Alternative to Hydroxychloroquine?" Dr. Joseph Mercola. April 28, 2020. Mercola.com.

"Is Wearing Three Masks Better than One?" An interview with Dr. Ted Noel. February 3, 2021. Mercola.com.

Jaws: The Story of a Hidden Epidemic. Sandra Kahn and Paul. R. Ehrlich. 2018. Stanford University Press.

"List of 21 Foods High in Iodine Content for Hypothyroidism." No author cited. September 15, 2019. Allremedies.com.

The Machinery of Life 2ⁿᵈ Edition. David S. Goodsell. 2009. Springer Science and Business Media, LLC.

"Magnesium and K2 Optimize Your Vitamin D Supplementation." Dr. Joseph Mercola. July 16, 2020. Mercola.com

"Magnesium by Nebulizer." Dr. Sarah Myhill. March 5, 2015. Drmyhill. co.uk.

"Magnesium: Nebulizing." Dr. Mark Sircus. www.DrSircus.com.

Magnesium: Reversing Disease. Thomas E. Levy, MD. 2019. MedFox Publishing.

"The Many Ways in Which Covid Vaccines May harm Your Health." Interview of Stephanie Seneff, PhD and Judy Mikovits, PhD. June 1, 2021. Mercola.com.

"Masks Likely Do Not Inhibit Viral Spread." Sn interview with Denis Rancout, PhD. December 1, 2020. Mercola.com.

"Mass Vaccination Triggers Spike in Cases, Deaths." Mike Whitney. June 2021. Mercola.com.

"'Medical Aspects and Applications of Humic Substances' Regarding the Antiviral Activity of Humic Substances." Dr. Renate Klocking and Dr. Bjorn Helbig. Friedrich Schiller University, Jena, Germany. Article available on SupremeFulvic.com.

"Medical Ignorance and the Mass Murder of Coronavirus Patients." W. Gifford-Jones, MD. October 20, 2020. Orthomolecular Medicine News Service.

"Microbiome and the Immune System: From a Healthy Steady State to Allergy Associated Disruption." Mezouar et al. October 24, 2018. Human Microbiome Journal.

Micro-Cosmos: Four Billion Years of Microbial Evolution. Lynn Margulis and Dorian Sagan. 1986. Summit Books.

The Mineral Fix: How to Optimize your Mineral Intake for Energy, Longevity, Immunity, Sleep, and More. Dr. James DiNicolantonio and Siim Land. 2021. Independently published.

Minerals: Key to Vibrant Health and Life Force. Jacob Swilling, PhD. 2003. Know Your Options Inc.

Miracles from the Vault: Anthology of Underground Cures. Jenny Thompson and Health Sciences Institute. 2013. Health Sciences Institute.

The Miraculous Properties of Ionized Water: The Definitive Guide to the World's Healthiest Substance. Bob McCauley. 2006. Spartan Enterprises, Inc.

"More Health Benefits of Quercetin Revealed." Dr. Joseph Mercola. January 26, 2020. Mercola.com

The Most Effective Natural Cures on Earth: The Surprising Unbiased Truth about What Treatments Work and Why. Jonny Bowden, PhD. 2008. Fair Winds Press.

"The Most Powerful Natural Antibiotics Known to Mankind." Bob. July 17, 2017. Askaprepper.com.

"Mutated COVID-19 Virus Marketed to Justify New Lockdowns." Dr. Joseph Mercola. January 7, 2021. Mercola.com.

"NAC in the Treatment of COVID-19." Roger Seheult. September 2020. MedCram Lecture.

Natural Allopathic Infectious Protocol : Dr. Marc Sircus, www. DrSircus.com

Natural Health Remedies: Your A-Z Blueprint for Vibrant Health. Janet Maccaro, PhD. 2006. Siloam, Strang Publishing Group.

Nature's Virus Killers. Mark Stengler, ND with Arden Moore. 2000. M. Evans and Company, Inc., New York.

"Nebulizing Magnesium and other Medicinals." Dr. Marc Sircus. www. DrSircus.com.

"Non-Pharmaceutical Infection Control." Dr. Marc Sircus. www. DrSircus.com.

The Nutraceutical Revolution. Richard Firshein, ND. 1998. Riverhead Books.

"Nutritional Strategies to Support your Immune System." No author cited. April 28, 2020. Linus Pauling Institute.

Nature's Robots: A History of Proteins. Charles Tanford and Jacqueline Reynolds. 2001. Oxford University Press.

"Newest MATH+ Protocol." An interview with Dr. Joseph Varon. August 3, 2021. Mercola.com.

Nutrient Power: Heal Your Biochemistry and Heal Your Brain. William J. Walsh, PhD. 2012. Skyhorse Publishing.

"Nutritional Adjuncts to the Fat-Soluble Vitamins." Christopher Masterjohn. January 28, 2013; Weston A. Price Foundation, wwwwestonaprice.org/author/masterjohn.

Nutrition, Health and Disease. Gary Price Todd, MD. 1985. Whitford Press.

"Nutrition to Treat and Prevent COVID-19." Dr. Y, Dr. Andrew W. Saul, and Robert G. Smith. January 17, 2021. Orthomolecular Medicine News Service.

"Nutrition's Dynamic Duos." Harvard Health Letter. July 2009. Harvard Health Publishing, Harvard Medical School.

"NY Doctor Proved Everyone Wrong about Hydroxychloroquine." An interview with Dr. Vladimir Zelenko. February 9, 2021. Mercola.com.

Olive Oil: Proven Benefits; Healthline.com, no author cited

Orthomolecular Medicine for Everyone: Megavitamin Therapeutics for Families and Physicians. Abram Hoffer, MD, PhD and Andrew W. Saul, PhD. 2008. Basic Health Publications.

The Oxygen Prescription: The Miracle of Oxidative Therapies. Nathaniel Altman. 1995. Healing Arts Press.

"Ozone Therapy for Coronavirus." Dr. Joseph Mercola. April 6, 2020. Mercola.com.

"Pandemic Virus Industrial Complex Is World's Greatest Threat." Dr. Joseph Mercola. June 20, 2021. Mercola.com.

"Pentagon-Funded Nonprofit Covering Up SARS-CoV-2 Origin." Dr. Joseph Mercola. January 7, 2021. Mercola.com.

"Pfizer's COVID-19 Pill Under Development Already Exists in Several Other Forms." Dr. M. Sircus. April 30, 2021. drsircus.com.

A Planet of Viruses. Carl Zimmer. 2011. University of Chicago.

Plague of Corruption: Restoring Faith in the Promise of Science (Children's Health Defense). by Dr. Judy Mikovits and Kent Heckenlively, Jr. 2020. Children's Health Defense.

Primal Panacea. Thomas E. Levy, MD. 2011. MedFox Publishing.

Probiotics: Protection against Infection; Using Nature's Tiny Warriors to Stem Infection and Fight Disease. Case Adams, PhD. 2012. Logical Books.

The Probiotics Revolution. Gary B. Huffnagle, PhD. 2007. Bantam Books.

"Protected Group Immunity, not a Vaccine, is the Way to Stop the COVID-19 Pandemic." by Richard Z. Cheng MD, PhD. April 30, 2020. Orthomolecular Medicine News Service.

"Published Research and Articles on Vitamin C as a Consideration for Pneumonia, Lung Infections, and the Novel Coronavirus" (SARS-CoV-2/COVID-19). Graham Player, PhD, Andrew W. Saul, Damien Dowling MBBS, MRSB, Gert Schuitemaiker, PhD. March 22, 2020. Orthomolecular Medicine News Service.

"Quercetin and Vitamin C: An Experimental, Synergistic Therapy for the Prevention and Treatment of Sars-CoV-2-related Disease (COVID-19)." Biancatelli, Berrill, Catravas, and Marik. June 19, 2020. Frontiers in Immunology.

"Quercetin and Vitamin D: Allies Against Coronavirus?" Joseph Mercola. March 16, 2020. Mercola.com.

Rapid Virus Recovery. Thomas E. Levy, MD, JD. MedFox Publishing 2021.

Rare Earths: Forbidden Cures. Joel D. Wallach, DVM and Ma Lan MD. 1994. Double Happiness Publishing Company.

"Resolving 'Long-Haul COVID' and Vaccine Toxicity: Neutralizing the Spike Protein." Dr. Thomas E. Levy. June 21, 2021. Orthomolecular News Service.

"A Review of Helpful Antiviral Strategies." An interview with Dr. Andrew Saul, Editor in chief of the Orthomolecular Medicine News Service. April 20, 2020. Mercola.com.

The Root of All Disease. E. G. Heinrich. Condensed version on SupremeFulvic.com.

"Sanitizing Your Nose?" Dr. Joseph Mercola. April 5, 2021. Mercola.com.

"Scientists Worry That Next Flu Season Will Be a Disaster." Dr. Joseph Mercola. June 29, 2021, Mercola.com.

"The Search for SARS-CoV-2's Origin Must Continue." Dr. Joseph Mercola. January 15, 2021. Mercola.com.

"Seniors Dying after COVID Vaccine Labeled as Natural Causes." Dr. Joseph Mercola. February 4, 2021. Mercola.com.

"Several COVID-19 Vaccines Are Made Using Aborted Fetal Cells." Dr. Joseph Mercola. December 21, 2020. Mercola.com.

"Simple Hacks That Make Fasting Easy." An interview with David Asprey. January 18, 2021. Mercola.com.

"Simple Strategies that Will Improve Your Immunity." Interview with Dr. James DiNicolantonio and Siim Land. December 7, 2020. Mercola.com.

Sleep to Save Your Life: The Complete Guide to Living Longer and Healthier through Restorative Sleep. Gerard T. Lombardo, MD. 2005. HarperCollins Publisher.

"Smothering the Fire: How Vitamin C Can Stop Viral Infections Quickly." Tom Taylor. May 28, 2020. Orthomolecular Medicine News Service.

Sodium Bicarbonate: Rich Man's, Poor Man's Cancer Treatment (eBook, second edition). Dr Marc Sircus. www.Dr.Sircus.com.

Solved: The Riddle of Illness; How Managing Your Thyroid Can Help You Fight and Control. Stephen E. Langer, MD and James F. Scheet. 1984. Keats Publishing, Inc.

"Sore Throat: Effective Treatment Means More Vitamins, Fewer Drugs." Ralph Campbell, MD. March 21, 2018. Orthomolecular Medicine News Service.

"Spike Protein Damages Vascular Cells." Dr. Joseph Mercola. May 26, 2021. Mercola.com.

Studies in Deficiency Disease. Robert McCarrison. 1921. Reprinted by Cornell University Library.

Successful High Dose Vitamin C Treatment of patients with Serious and Critical COVID-19 Infection: by Richard Cheng, M.D. Ph.D., March 18,2020; Orthomolecular Medicine News Service

Survival of the Sickest: The Surprising Connections between Disease and Longevity. Dr. Sharon Moalem. 2007. HarperCollins Books.

"Today's Greatest Alternative Medicines." Compiled by the Health Sciences Research Team. 2009. Health Sciences Institute.

The Truth about Contagion: Exploring Theories about How Disease Spreads. Thomas S. Cowan, MD and Sally Fallon Morell. 2021. Skyhorse Publishing.

"The Truth about COVID-19 'Long Haulers.'" Dr. Joseph Mercola. November 24, 2020. Mercola.com.

"The Truth about Taking Zinc Lozenges for Colds." Frank Shallenberger MD. July 25, 2018. www.advancedbionutritionals.com.

Trace Elements and Man: Some Positive and Negative Aspects. Henry A. Schroeder, MD. 1973. Devin Adair Company .

Treasury of Natural Cures. Dr. Jonathan V. Wright. 2013. NewMarket Health Publishing.

"The Treatment of Infectious Disease Using Vitamin C and Other Nutrients." Margot Desbois. January 20, 2021. Orthomolecular Medicine News Service.

"Types of Influenza Viruses." Center for Disease Control and Prevention. No date given. CDC website.

The Underground Health Reporter: Little Known Discoveries that Make a Dramatic Impact on Your Health by Underground Health Reporter. Various authors. 2009. Think-Outside-of-the-Book Publishers

Unreported Truths about COVID-19 and Lockdowns: Part 1 Introduction and Death Counts and Estimates. Alex Berenson. June 2020. Bowker Publishing.

Unreported Truths about COVID-19 and Lockdowns: Part 2 Update and Examination of Lockdowns as a Strategy: Alex Berenson. August 2020. Bowker Publishing.

Unreported Truths about COVID-19 and Lockdowns: Part 3 Masks. Alex Berenson. November 2020. Bowker Publishing.

Unreported Truths about COVID-19 and Lockdowns: Part 4 Vaccines. Alex Berenson. March 2021. Bowker Publishing.

"Vaccination: What's Trust Got to Do with It?" Barbara Loe Fisher. September 25, 2020. Mercola.com.

"Vaccine Effectiveness: How Well Do the Flu Vaccines Work?" Center for Disease Control and Prevention. No date given. CDC website.

"Vaccine Insider: COVID-19 Mass Vaccination Campaign Must End." An interview with Geert Vanden Bossche, PhD. March 30, 2021. Mercola.com.

Viruses and the Evolution of Life. Luis P. Villarreal. 2005. The American Society of Microbiology Press.

The Virusphere: From Common Colds to Ebola Epidemics; Why We Need the Viruses that Plague Us. Frank Ryan. 2020. Prometheus Books.

"Vitamin A Treatment for Measles." Committee on Infectious Disease. May 5, 1993. *Pediatrics*, Volume 91.

"Vitamin C, Titrating to Bowel Tolerance, Anascorbemia, and Acute Induced Scurvy." Robert F. Cathcart III, MD. 1981. Medical Hypotheses.

"Vitamin C and Coronavirus: Not a Vaccine, Just a Humble Cure." William F. Simmons and Robert G. Smith, PhD. May 4, 2020. Orthomolecular Medicine News Service.

"Vitamin C and COVID-19 Coronavirus." Damien Downing, MBBS, MRSB and Gert Schuitemaker, PhD. February 28, 2020. Orthomolecular Medicine News Service.

"Vitamin C Protects against Coronavirus." Dr. Andrew W. Saul. January 26, 2020. Orthomolecular Medicine News Service.

"Vitamin C Treatment for COVID-19 Being Silenced." An interview with Dr. Andrew Saul, editor in chief of the Orthomolecular Medicine News Service. December 14, 2020. Mercola.com.

"Vitamin C Works for Sepsis. Will it Work for Coronavirus?" Dr. Joseph Mercola. March 2, 2020. Mercola.com.

"Vitamin D3 versus D2." Dr. Joseph Mercola. March 25, 2018. Mercola.com.

The Vitamin D Cure. James E. Dowd, MD and Diane Stafford. 2009. John Wiley and Sons, Inc.

"Vitamin D Cuts SARS-CoV-2 Infection Rate by Half." Dr. Joseph Mercola. September 29, 2020. Mercola.com.

"Vitamin D Deficiency as a Cause of Disease and Safe High Dose Vitamin D Treatments." Dr. Marc Sircus. August 2, 2019. www.DrSircus.com.

"Vitamin D Protects against Colds, Flu, finds Major Global Study." University of Queen Mary, London. February 16, 2017. Science Daily.

The Vitamin D Revolution: How the Power of this Amazing Vitamin Can Change Your Life. Soram Khalsa, MD. 2009. Hay House, Inc.

"Vitamin D Saves Lives." Prof. Keith Scott-Mumby. July 1, 2020. Alternative-doctor.com.

"Vitamin D Supplementation Reduces COVID-19 Deaths by 64%." Dr. Joseph Mercola. June 23, 2021. Mercola.com.

"Vitamin D Supplements Could Reduce Risk of Influenza and COVID-19 Infection and Death." William B. Grant, PhD and Carole A Baggerly. April 9, 2020. Orthomolecular Medicine News Service.

"Vitamin E." Mayo Clinic staff. November 13, 2020. Mayoclinic.org.

The Vitamins: Fundamental Aspects in Nutrition and Health, Fourth Edition. Gerald. F. Combs Jr. 2012. Academic Press Publishers.

Water and Life: The Unique Properties of H20. Edited by Ruth M. Lynden-Bell, Simon Conway Morris, John D. Barrow, John L. Finney, and Charles L. Harper Jr. 2012. CRC Press.

"Why Children Should Not Receive the Covid Shot." Peter Doshi, PhD. June 10, 2021. Public hearing by the US Food and Drug Administration's Vaccines and Related Biological Products Advisory Committee.

The Wonderful World within You: Understanding Your Individual Differences Can Be the Key to a Healthier More Vigorous Life. Dr. Roger J. Williams. 1998. Bio Communication Press.

Your Natural Medicine Cabinet: A Practical Guide to Drug-Free Remedies for Common Ailments. Burke Lennihan. 2012. Green Healing Press.

"Zinc Ionophore Activity of Quercetin and Epigallocatechin-gallate: From Hepa 1-6 Cells to a Liposome Model." H. Dabbagh-Bazarbachi et al. 2014. Journal of Agricultural Food Chemistry.

"Zinc is Key for COVID-19 Treatment and Prevention." Dr. Joseph Mercola. October 30, 2020. Mercola.com.

"Zinc Supplementation and COVID-19." July 17, 2020. National Institutes of Health website.

"Zn 2+ Inhibits Coronavirus and Arterivirus RNA Polymerase Activity in Vitro and Zinc Ionophores Block the Replication of These Viruses in Cell Culture." A. W. Veithuis et al. May17, 2010. PLoS pathogens. www. Plospathogens.org.

ABOUT THE AUTHOR

Dr. Ralph La Guardia has spent over three decades researching alternative ways of treating and preventing diseases of all types. He has been in private practice in Connecticut for more than thirty years. During that time, he has learned what alternative and natural methods work and which ones are "snake oil." He has read hundreds of books and research articles on alternative ways of treating different diseases and has a huge personal library of many of these out-of-print books. He is well known in the medical underground of pioneering integrative medical practitioners. Integrative medicine is the highly effective combination of traditional and alternative medicine. He has authored the *The Doomsday Book of Medicine*, considered by many to be the best book on medical prepping. He has also written *The Bible of Alternative Medicine*. He lives on an organic farm in Connecticut with his lovely wife Lynne, his feisty ninety-one-year-old mother Mary, and their three dogs and four horses. When not practicing medicine or writing, he spends most of his time in his orchards or his geodesic dome greenhouse, experimenting with growing and propagating edible fruits of all kinds.